Developments in Gastroenterology

VOLUME 13

The titles published in this series are listed at the end of this volume.

COELIAC DISEASE

40 years gluten-free

edited by

M. L. MEARIN
Department of Paediatrics,
University Hospital,
Leiden, The Netherlands

and

C. J. J. MULDER
Department of Hepato-gastroenterology,
Rijnstate Hospital,
Arnhem, The Netherlands

KLUWER ACADEMIC PUBLISHERS
DORDRECHT / BOSTON / LONDON

ISBN 0-7923-1160-4

Published by Kluwer Academic Publishers,
P.O. Box 17, 3300 AA Dordrecht, The Netherlands.

Kluwer Academic Publishers incorporates
the publishing programmes of
D. Reidel, Martinus Nijhoff, Dr W. Junk and MTP Press.

Sold and distributed in the U.S.A. and Canada
by Kluwer Academic Publishers,
101 Philip Drive, Norwell, MA 02061, U.S.A.

In all other countries, sold and distributed
by Kluwer Academic Publishers Group,
P.O. Box 322, 3300 AH Dordrecht, The Netherlands.

Printed on acid-free paper

Printed in the Netherlands

TABLE OF CONTENTS

NOTE OF THE EDITORS:

In the text all the gamma ( ) symbols have been substitued by tau (τ).

COELIAC DISEASE:

40 YEARS GLUTEN-FREE.

On the 30th of May 1950 the Dutch paediatrician Dicke published his thesis on the effect of gluten on coeliac patients. However on the 24th of November 1940 Dicke introduced his gluten-free diet in Amsterdam to the Dutch Pediatric Society, 50 years ago.

As a result of the work of Dicke, the gluten-free diet as standard treatment for coeliac disease was discovered. To commemorate this performance an International Symposium on Coeliac Disease was organized in Leiden on 22th May 1990, under the auspices of the Dutch Coeliac Society.

It is now known that in genetically predisposed individuals certain gliadin peptides can produce alterations in the small intestine which recover on a gluten-free diet. The mechanism by which gliadin produces damage of the small intestine and the eventual immunological mechanisms implicated in the disease are still obscure. The relationship between coeliac disease and malignancy and the possible protective effect of the gluten-free diet means that new techniques which are able to detect small amounts of gluten in food are necessary.

This book contains the proceedings of this international symposium that brought together almost 250 participants from 25 countries. Research on coeliac disease can only be hampered by the lack of research funds, but not by lack of research topics.

We hope that this symposium-book will allow up-to-date information exchange between investigators and clinicians, and will stimulate investigators to contribute their data to literature.

Luisa Mearin
Chris Mulder

M.L. Mearin, Dept. Paediatrics, University Hospital,
PO Box 9600, 2300 RC, Leiden, The Netherlands.

C.J.J. Mulder, Dept. Hepato-Gastroenterology, Rijnstate Hospital,
PO Box 9555, 6800 TA, Arnhem, The Netherlands.

M. L. Mearin and C. J. J. Mulder (eds.), Coeliac Disease, ix–x.

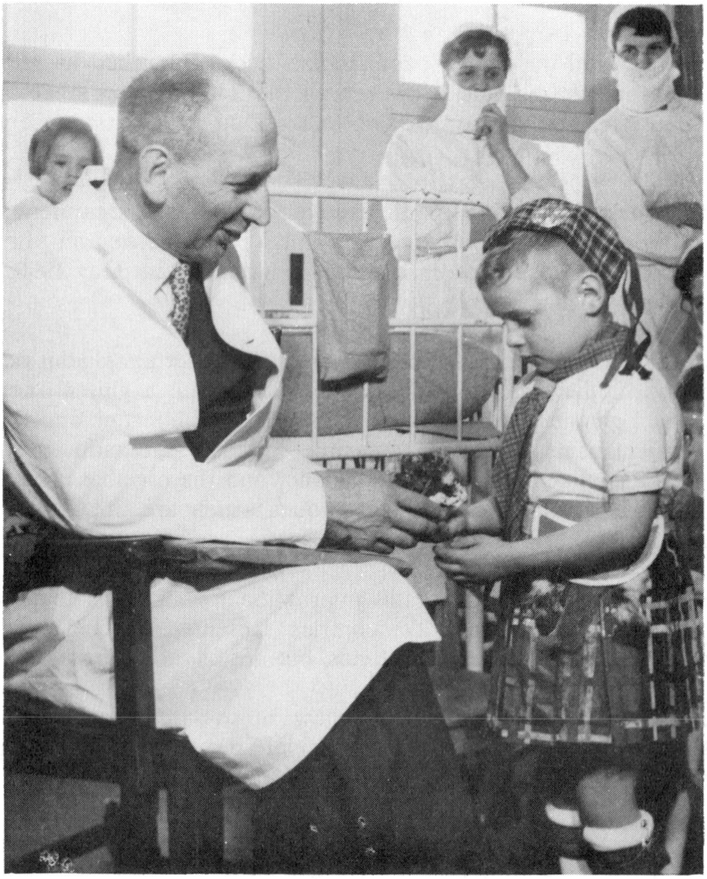

1950 - 1990 40 YEARS GLUTEN-FREE

COELIAKIE

EEN ONDERZOEK NAAR DE NADELIGE INVLOED VAN SOMMIGE GRAANSOORTEN OP DE LIJDER AAN COELIAKIE

★

COELIAC DISEASE

INVESTIGATION OF THE HARMFUL EFFECTS OF CERTAIN TYPES OF CEREAL ON PATIENTS WITH COELIAC DISEASE

(WITH SUMMARY IN ENGLISH)

PROEFSCHRIFT

TER VERKRIJGING VAN DE GRAAD VAN DOCTOR IN DE GENEESKUNDE AAN DE RIJKSUNIVERSITEIT TE UTRECHT, OP GEZAG VAN DEN RECTOR MAGNIFICUS DR. H. J. M. WEVE, HOOGLERAAR IN DE FACULTEIT DER GENEESKUNDE, VOLGENS BESLUIT VAN DE SENAAT DER UNIVERSITEIT IN HET OPENBAAR TE VERDEDIGEN OP DINSDAG 30 MEI 1950, DES NAMIDDAGS 4 UUR

DOOR

WILLEM KAREL DICKE

GEBOREN TE DORDRECHT

HISTORY OF COELIAC DISEASE. DICKE AND THE ORIGIN OF THE GLUTEN-FREE DIET.

A.S. Peña. Department of Gastroenterology, Leiden University Hospital. PO Box 9600, 2300 RC, Leiden, The Netherlands.

In 1988 Dr. Paveley published a succinct history of coeliac disease (CD). One of the historical landmarks of CD has been the discovery that a component of a normal diet, wheat, is toxic to the coeliac patient. Dicke in collaboration with Van de Kamer and Weijers in Utrecht, demonstrated this with careful experiments performed on patients during different periods using different cereals. In his assay, Dr. Paveley quotes a lecture delivered by Sir Christopher Booth to the Derby Medical Society in November 1983. According to Booth the idea of the wheat-free diet occurred to Dicke during the Second World War when there was a shortage of bread, although Dicke first noticed a possible relationship between wheat and a condition of malabsorption with a rash in a child in 1930. Several months after the publication of the article by Dr. Paveley, Dr. Smits challenged the story that the wartime food availability has had any effect on Dicke's idea which led to his discovery, as Dicke had already made observations leading to the gluten-free diet on children born before, and during the beginning of the war. He further added: "Sir Christopher Booth has enjoyed the tale as it makes a nice story, but I do not think there is any evidence whatsoever to support it". After consulting several sources, the story can be summarized as follows: In Chapter III of Dicke's thesis, entitled: "Treatment with a wheat-free diet" he stated that the origin of his idea on this kind of dietary treatment was an observation of ME van Dusseldorp and HA Stheeman during the treatment of a coeliac patient. He then quotes a passage of the publication by Stheeman in 1932. Stheeman reports 4 cases of CD in children. He concentrated his message on the significant improvement on the coeliac children with Ventraemon, a powder, from stomach mucosa, which due to its bad taste was administered on bread (!), with jam or sugar. However, Dicke was particularly interested in case 3 "One child who had three severe episodes of diarrhoea while in hospital. Each time he had bread. A single Dutch rusk (biscuit) was enough to cause him a collapse". Mrs. Dicke has recently informed us that during the German occupation, Dicke, at the time the Director of the Juliana Children's Hospital in The Hague, ordered tulip bulbs to supplement the hospital food, since there was not enough to eat. Occasionally, the children had Dutch rusks and the coeliac children became ill. Dicke was then convinced that wheat had to be the offending agent for these children. Dicke had another chance to reconfirm his conclusion when Allied aircraft came (operation Manna) and dropped Swedish white bread over occupied Holland and coeliac children became ill again. This was discussed during the weekly meeting with Prof. Mulder and Dr. Haex at the Leiden University Hospital. Dicke was a member of the Board of Directors of the University of Leiden, before he went to Utrecht.

INTRODUCTION

In 1988 Dr. Paveley (1) published in the British Medical Journal a beautiful

M. L. Mearin and C. J. J. Mulder (eds.), Coeliac Disease, 3–7.

succinct history of coeliac disease, from the first clinical descriptions to the introduction of peroral intestinal biopsy. One of the historical landmarks of coeliac disease has been the discovery that a component of a normal diet, wheat, is toxic to the coeliac patient. Dicke (2) demonstrated this with careful experiments performed on patients during different periods using different cereals. Several factors contributed to transform this clinical observation into a scientifically proven fact. First, J.H. van de Kamer from the Central Institute for Nutrition Research in Utrecht had developed an accurate method to measure faecal fats (3,4). Then, H.A. Weijers from the Wilhelmina Children's Hospital, permitted the correct measurement of faecal fat excretion of children with coeliac disease during different dietary regimes by using the excretion coefficient of saturated and non-saturated faecal fats (5). However, it is clear from reading Dicke's thesis as well as the publication of van de Kamer (6), that when Dicke went to Utrecht to perform the crucial experiments which were described in his thesis under the leadership of Professor ten Bokkel Huinnik, he already knew that wheat was the offending substance for coeliac patients.

In his assay on the history of coeliac disease, Dr. Paveley quotes a lecture delivered some years ago by Sir Christopher Booth in which he has said that the idea of the wheat-free diet came to Dicke during the "hunger" winter of the Second World War: -"Another more important shortage occurred during the war. In The Netherlands there was a scarcity of bread and, according to Sir Christopher Booth (In a lecture to the Derby Medical Society in November 1983), Dicke, a Dutch paediatrician, observed that the so called "coeliac sprue" diminished remarkably during this shortage. Apparently Dicke first noticed a possible relationship between wheat and a "condition of malabsorption with a rash in a young child in 1930".

Several months after the publication of the article by Dr. Paveley, Dr. Smits (7) challenged this view. According to him, the story about the wartime food availability having had any effect whatsoever on allowing Dicke to come to his conclusions, was not true: -"I was again interested to read Sir Christopher Booth's notion that Dr Dicke's observations were that coeliac disease diminished remarkably during the war in The Netherlands because of the shortage of wheat and hence bread. In my view this observation is spurious". He further added that Sir Christopher Booth has enjoyed the tale as it makes a nice story but he does not think there is any evidence whatsoever to support it. Sir Christopher Booth (8) replied that he talked to Dicke before he died -"He was quite clear in his conversation with me that it was a young mother's statement that her coeliac child's rash improved if she removed bread from the diet that first alerted his interest. This was when he was a paediatrician in the Hague in 1936".

AIM OF THE PRESENT ARTICLE AND SOURCES CONSULTED

To commemorate the 40th anniversary of the publication of Dicke's thesis with "The Dicke symposium" it was decided to review this aspect of the history of coeliac disease. Since Dicke, van de Kamer and Weijers are not alive, I have consulted some of Dr. Dicke's articles, contemporaneous publications, visited Mrs. A. Dicke-Schouten, his widow, and Prof. A.J.Ch. Haex, former Professor of Gastroenterology at Leiden and former President of The Netherlands Society of Gastroenterology. Prof. Haex conceived the idea of instituting a Dicke Medal to honour fundamental pioneering work in gastroenterology. He was, to a great extent, responsible for honouring Dicke with the first Dicke's gold medal and later during the celebrations of the 60th Anniversary of the Foundation of the Netherlands Society for Gastroenterology, the Dicke gold medal was awarded to Sir Christopher Booth for his pioneer work in the absorption of Vitamin B12 and his contributions to research on the small intestine, gastroenterology in general and medical history (9).

THE HISTORY OF THE WHEAT-FREE DIET ACCORDING TO DICKE

Dicke left two written accounts about the origin of the gluten-free diet. One, in his Thesis (2), read at the University of Utrecht on the 30th of May 1950. He clearly stated in Chapter III concerning the origin of the treatment with a wheat-free diet:- "An observation made by M.E. van Dusseldorp and H.A. Stheeman, during the treatment of a coeliac child was the origin of this diet". He also quotes a publication by H.A. Stheeman (10). This article was based on a presentation held during a meeting in The Hague on the 19th of May 1932 and was published in the Netherlands Journal of Medicine on Saturday the 15th of october 1932. A report of 4 cases of coeliac disease in children is given. These children were treated with 10 g. daily of Ventraemon (Homogenized stomach powder) with excellent results. Curiously, Dr. Stheeman remarked that :-"Ventraemon has a very bad taste. It was, therefore, given on **bread** with jam or in a kind of yoghurt mixed with some sugar. It completely disguises the bad taste". However, Dicke's attention was directed to Case 3.: "T.F. had been admitted for the second time to the Juliana Children's Hospital. He was admitted for the first time at the age of 19 months in an appalling condition of malnourishment. During his stay in the hospital he has had diarrhoea three times. At one time he lost 1½ kg in weight. Every time, these relapses had been preceded by the consumption of wheat flour. He showed a definite idiosyncracy against biscuit, bread and flour. The ingestion of only one biscuit had once caused a collapse". The other written reference to the wheat-free diet given by Dicke, probably the first written account of this diet, was based on a communication to The Dutch Pediatric Society delivered by Dicke on Sunday 24th of November 1940 in Amsterdam. The proceedings were published in the Netherlands Journal of Medicine on Saturday the 19th of April 1941 (11). W.K. Dicke, A simple diet for the Gee-Herter Syndrome: "In recent literature is stated that the diet of Haas (bananas) and Fanconi (fruit) give the best results in the treatment of patients suffering from the above mentioned syndrome. At present, these items are not available, therefore, I give a simple diet, which is helping the children during this time of rationing"...."The diet should not have any bread. Some biscuits are sometimes tolerated. A hot meal twice a day is also tolerated. The third meal can be sweet or sour porridge (without wheat flour)". After the presentation, Mrs. Stärcke-Polenaar asks if rye bread is tolerated. Dicke says, he has not yet tried it. It is clear that in 1940 Dicke knew that wheat was the main offending element of the diet. Ten years later in collaboration with Weijers and van de Kamer he was able to show that wheat and rye contained the offending agent.

SOME NOTES ON THE PAEDIATRICIAN DICKE

Dicke was born on 15th of February 1905. He was trained in the Juliana Children's Hospital in The Hague. Mrs. A. Dicke-Schouten remembers that during this time he once made a diagnosis of erythema nodosum in a child with a characteristic rash. This impressed Dr. Stheeman, who was the Director of the Hospital. When Dicke finished his studies, Dr. Stheeman, asked him to come to the Juliana Children's Hospital for his training in paediatrics and to work with him. Dicke followed his advice, finished the training and became Chef de Clinique when Mrs. van Dusseldorp succeeded Dr. Stheeman as probably the first female Director of a hospital in The Netherlands. Mrs. Dicke informed us that Mrs. van Dusseldorp died at a young age of pneumoccocal peritonitis, a condition diagnosed by Dicke. He succeeded her as Medical Director of the Juliana Children's Hospital at the age of 31. He continued to be interested in children with coeliac disease, although, he also had an interest in pulmonary disease, after having acquired pulmonary tuberculosis from a sick child (12).

During the German invasion he moved the in-patients to another village. Mrs Dicke remained with her two children in the hospital which was surrounded by the German soldiers. Dicke ordered tulip bulbs to supplement the hospital food, since there were not enough cereals. Remarkably as Dicke commented "To the coeliac children, the shortage of food was less severe than the toxic effects of wheat products" (13). Occasionally, the children received Dutch rusks (beschuit). Dicke was convinced then that the wheat was the offending agent for the coeliac children. Consequently he forbade to give them wheat products. When the English and American aircraft came with the Swedish white bread (13) he had another chance to reconfirm his conclusion, as Dicke told Dr. Haex and Prof. Mulder during their weekly meetings at the Leiden University Hospital. Dicke was on the Board of Directors of the University of Leiden, before he took the chair of Paediatrics in Utrecht. From 1945 to 1948 while Dicke was in the Hague, he continued to treat coeliac children and some adults who had heard of the good results with a wheat-free diet. From July 1948 till January 1950, four children in the Wilhelmina Children's Hospital in Utrecht and one in the Juliana Children's Hospital in The Hague were challenged with different cereals under a precise protocol to measure the amount of faeces, faecal fat, and the fat absorption coefficient. On the 30th May 1950 Dicke successfully defended the following conclusions: "The cause of the phenomena: (a) anorexia, (b) increased amount of faeces; (c) increased excretion of fat, is unknown, but they are elicited or aggravated by certain types of flour, especially wheat and rye flours. Wheat starch, the effect of which was studied, does not give rise to these phenomena. This is proof that the harmful factor must be situated in a component of wheat flour other than the starch" (2).

IMMEDIATE AND LONG-TERM REPERCUSSION OF DICKE'S OBSERVATION

Dicke's observations opened a new era in the treatment of childhood coeliac disease. The Dutch observations were soon confirmed in Scandinavia (14,15), England (16) and Germany (17). The treatment of adult coeliac disease took some years to start. First with case reports in Canada (18), The United States (19), The Netherlands (20), and it was not until 1957 that French (21) published a series of 22 patients. Recent studies in England suggest that the gluten-free diet protects the coeliac patient against the development of malignancy (22). If this is confirmed there is no doubt that Dicke's clinical observation will reach areas he never dreamed of.

REFERENCES

1 Paveley WF. From Areteus to Crosby: A history of coeliac disease. Br Med J 1988;297:1646-9.
2 Dicke WK. Coeliac disease. Investigation of the harmful effects of certain types of cereal on patients with coeliac disease. Thesis, Utrecht 1950.
3 Kamer JH van de. Vet in Faeces. De gehaltebepaling en de bepaling van het moleculair gewicht, in verband met de vetresorptie van de mens. Proefschrift Utrecht 1948.
4 Kamer JH van de, ten Bokkel Huinink,H, en Weijers HA. Rapid method for the determination of fat in feces. J Biol Chem 1949;177:347- 55.
5 Weijers HA. De vetresorptie van gezonde en zieke zuigelingen en kinderen in het bijzonder van coeliakiepatiënten. Thesis, Utrecht 1950.
6 Kamer van de JH. Coeliac disease, sprue syndrome and the metabolism of fat. A review of papers by Dicke, Frazer, Van de kamer, Tegelaers, Trap and Weijers. Voeding 1952;13:1-21.
7 Smits BJ. History of coeliac disease. Br Med J 1989; 298:387.
8 Booth CC. History of coeliac disease. Br Med J 1989; 298:527.
9 Haex AJCh. Address given on the occasion of the awarding of the Dicke Gold Medal to Prof. CC Booth on behalf of The Netherlands Society for Gastroenterology, at Woudschoten on the 26th of October 1973.
10 Stheeman HA. De intestinale infantilismus en zijn behandeling met Ventraemon. N T Geneesk 1932;76: 4823-41.
11 Dicke WK. Eenvoudig dieet bij het syndroom van Gee-Herter. N T Geneesk 1941;85:1715-6.
12 Streef AM, Dicke WK. De behandeling van het pleura-empyeembij kinderen. Overzicht van vijtig gevallen. N T Genesk 1941;85:323-31.
13 Haex AJCh. Het bestaansrecht van de Gastro-Enterologie binnen de interne Geneeskunde. Openbare Les 15 December 1959. De Erven f. Bohn N.V. Haarlem. Pag. 13, 1959.
14 Scheepmaker N. Het Zweedse wittebrood. Erven thomas Rap, Vijverhof, Baarn, 1979.
15 Söderhjelm AL. Dietbehandlingen vid coeliaki.Nordisk Medicin 1952;10;Bd47:479-81.
16 Anderson CM, Frazer AC, French JM, Gerrard JW, Sammons HG, Smellie JM. Coeliac disease: Gastro-intestinal studies and the effect of dietary wheat flour. Lancet 1952;i:836-42.
17 Krainick HG, Debatin F. Der Schädliche mehleffekt bei der kindlichen cöliakie. Klin Wochenschr 1953;31:958-9.
18 McIver C. Gluten-free diet in idiopathic steatorrhoea. Report of a case. Lancet 1952;ii:1112-4.
19 Ruffin JM, Carter DD, Johnston DH, Baylin GJ. "Wheat-free" diet in the treatment of Sprue. N Eng J med 1954; 250:281-2.
20 Haex AJCh, Lips JB. Nieuwe mogelijkheden bij de behandeling van Spruw. Ned Tijdsch Geneesk 1955;99: 102-6.
21 French JM, Hawkins CF, Smith N. The effect of a wheat-gluten-free diet in adult idiopathic steatorrhoea. A study of 22 cases. Quart J Med 1957,26:481-99.
22 Holmes GKT, Prior P, Lane MR, Dope D, Allan RN. Malignancy in coeliac disease - effect of a gluten free diet. Gut 1989;30:333-8.

HLA AND COELIAC DISEASE, A FINNISH FAMILY STUDY

S. Koskimies, V. Lipsanen, M. Mäki*, J. Visakorpi*. Finnisch Red Cross Blood Transfusion Service, Tissue Typing Laboratory, Helsinki, Finland, *Department of Pediatrics, University Hospital of Tampere, Finland.

We have 36 families with coeliac disease (CD) included in our study. Altogether 163 persons were studied comprising 36 patients, 55 siblings of which 11 were HLA identical, 27 haploidentical and 17 non-identical to the patient and 72 parents. For all individuals a small bowel biopsy was performed. Serological HLA typing of HLA A, B and DR antigens were done on all individuals. RFLP analysis using DRB, DQA, DPA and DPB gene specific probes together with various restriction enzymes was done on 30 families. The frequency of DR3 antigen was increased as expected, 34 of 36 patients had this allele, two patients lacking DR3 had DR7 allele. 56% of the siblings had DR3 allele. DR1 frequency was strongly decreased among the patients, 3.3%, when it was present in 20% of the healthy siblings. RFLP of DQA gene studied with TaqI enzyme revealed a fragment of 4.8 kb in size which was present in 96.7% of the patients and in 62.9% of the patient haplotypes, when it was only in 30% of the sibling haplotypes. When DQB RFLP was analysed with PstI, a 5.2 kb fragment was found to be present in all patients but only in 24.7% of the unrelated controls. This fragment was found to be derived from both DR3 and DR7 positive haplotypes. None of the DPA TaqI fragments and DBP MspI fragments did strongly correlate to the disease. We conclude that DQ genes have the strongest association to the CD, DQB gene being the most primary associating gene, but DQA contributes to the penetration of the disease.

INTRODUCTION

CD is characterized by small intestine mucosal injury and malabsorption of most nutritients. Disease is activated by the ingestion of wheat gluten and similar proteins. The etiology and pathogenesis of the disease is not fully understood but it is thought that gluten induces an immunologically mediated intestinal damage in genetically predisposed individuals. Susceptibility to CD is strongly associated with some HLA genes, particularly with HLA-B8, DR3, DR7 and DQw2 alleles (1-5). Eighty to 90% of CD patients of Nothern European ancestry have the DR3 and DQw2 serologic specificities, however those markers are present also in over 20% of the healthy population. In Southern Europe the HLA - DR7 alleles has also been associated with CD (6). DR7 positive haplotypes often carry also DQw2 specificity like DR3 positive haplotypes do, suggesting that a DQ locus might most contribute to the susceptibility. Recent data obtained using PCR typing have been interpreted as suggesting that DQw2 and/or DP antigens are involved in CD susceptibility (7).
We have studied HLA-Class II genes among Finnish coeliac patients and their healthy family members and our results show that 100% association could be found with a particular DQB gene among the Finnish patients. DQA gene, however, contributes to the susceptibility too. No strong association with DP locus could be found.

M. L. Mearin and C. J. J. Mulder (eds.), Coeliac Disease, 9–13.

METHODS

Thirty one Finnish coeliac patients and their healthy family members entered this study. The diagnosis was based on the finding of total or subtotal villous atrophy on proximal jejunum and of normalization of the villous architecture together with disappearance of symptoms on gluten free diet. Alle healthy family members had jejunal biopsy too. HLA-typing for class I antigens was performed serologically using antibody mediated cytoxicity test. DR typing was performed serologically for alleles DR1-8, DRB, DQA, DQB, DPA and DPB genes were studied by analysing the restriction fragment lenght polymorphism (RFLP) using cDNA probes from the 10th Internatiol Histocompatibility workshop. Enzymes TaqI, PstI and MspI were used as indicated in the text together with Southern blot assay.

RESULTS AND DISCUSSION

The HLA-DR frequencies of the patients are compared to those of the random Finnish population and are presented in table I. It shows that CD is strongly associated with DR3, among the Finnish patients. No significant association was found with DR7 allele. Only 3 patients were negative for DR3 allele, having the phenotype DR7.6 and DR7.4. Six patients were homozygous for DR3, six were heterozygous for DR3/DR7 and none were homozygous for DR7.

TABLE I DR ALLELE FREQUENCIES IN COELIAC PATIENTS AND UNRELATED CONTROLS

	Patients (N=31) %	Controls (N=81) %
DR	3.3	38.3 *
DR2	13.3	30.9
DR3	90.3 +	17.3 *
DR3.1	86.7	17.3 *
DR3.2	6.7	1.2
DR4	16.7	34.6
DR5	6.7	9.9
DR6	20.0	22.2
DR7.1	10.0	3.7
DR7.2	16.7	14.8
DR8	3.3	12.3
DR10	-	1.2
DR3/3	20.0	3.7
DR3/7	20.0	2.5
DR7/7	-	-

DR7,6; DR7,4; DR7,6

(RFLP, TaqI) * = $p < 0.0005$
+ = DR3 negative patients

In table II the DR gene frequencies among the patients and their family members are shown. Of 62 patients 36 expressed the DR3 allele meanwhile only 15 of 62 siblings expressed the DR3 allele. Interestingly the DR7.2 positive haplotypes were present in a higher frequency among the healthy siblings than in the patients. Only 37% of the patients haplotypes belonged to the extended haplotypes group B8-DR3-DQw2-DPw1 (data not shown). In some populations this haplotype has been found in over 90% of the coeliac patients (8) while less than 70% of our patients had this haplotype.

TABLE II DR GENE FREQUENCIES IN 31 FAMILIES WITH COELIAC PATIENT

	Patients % (62 haplotypes)	Parents % (116 haplotypes)	Siblings % (62 haplotypes)
DR1	1.6	9.5	12.9
DR2	6.5	12.1	11.3
DR3.1	54.8	35.3	22.6
DR3.2	3.2	2.6	1.6
DR4	8.1	10.3	11.3
DR5	3.2	3.4	3.2
DR6	8.1	11.2	16.1
DR7.1	4.8	2.6	1.6
DR7.2	8.1	8.6	14.5
DR8	1.6	4.3	4.8

RFLP analysis was performed in DQA and DQB genes of 30 patients using TaqI and PstI enzymes respectively. A fragment of 4.8 kb in size picked up by DQA specific probe of TaqI digested DNA was found in 29 of 30 patients and only in 27.2% of the controls (Table III). PstI RFLP analysis of DQB gene revealed a 100% association with CD, only 24.7% of the controls had this marker gene.

TABLE III HLA-DQA AND DQB RFLP MARKERS IN COELIAC PATIENTS, FAMILY MEMBERS AND CONTROLS

	DQA- TaqI 4.8 kb	DQB PstI 5.2 kb
Patients (30)	96.7 % *	100.0 %
Healthy siblings (29)	65.5 %	68.9 %
Parents (58)	67.2 %	70.6 %
Controls (81)	27.2 %	24.7 %

* $p < 0.001$

The frequency of both markers was increased among the healthy family members also. Both markers were present in 96.5% of the patients, 60.3% of the parents and 51.0% of the siblings. Haplotypes positive for both markers were analysed. Such haplotypes were found in 54.3% of the patients' haplotypes, but only 33.6% and 25.8% of the parents' and siblings' haplotypes. None of the siblings were homozygous for such haplotypes while 17.2% of the patients were homozygous for both markers suggesting that DQ genes have also a dose effect on susceptibility to CD (Fig. I).

FIGURE I

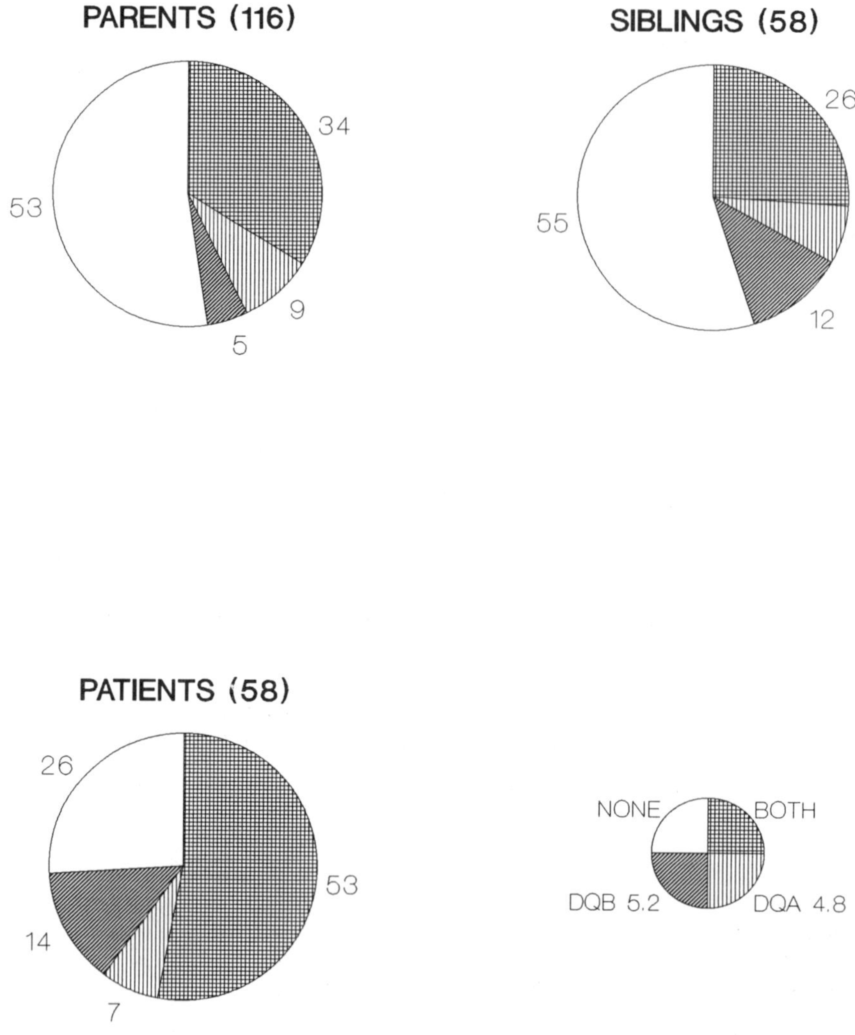

Three patients were negative for DR3 allele but positive for DR7, two had the subtype DR7.2 and one with DR7.2. All these patients had the DQB marker gene with PstI 5.2 kb fragment in DR7 positive haplotype but did not have the DQA TagI 4.8 kb marker on that haplotype. Two of these patients, however, had that DQA marker gene in the opposite chromosome carrying DR6 allele. DPA or DPB gene analysis did not show any strong correlation to the CD among the Finnish patients. Our results show that the DQB gene has the strongest effect on the susceptibility to CD but DQA has also a great impact to it. Only one patient was lacking the DQA marker gene. These marker genes were present either in cis or trans position thus suggesting that an antigen binding molecule comprising of α and β chains coded by DQA and DQB genes can be formed either as a product of maternal, paternal or both chromosomes. This is in agreement with the results of Sollid (5) and Lundin (11) and we could confirm it by haplotype analysis. It has been suggested that DP locus could be an additional risk factor in CD (9,10). DPw1 allele is in strong linkage disequilibrium in the extended haplotype B8-DR3-DQw2. Among the Finnish patients only less than 40% of the haplotypes belonged to this group. We could not show any strong association to DPA or DPB gene polymorphism thus suggesting that the association found in other populations reflect rather the strong linkage of DP to DR3 and DQw2 than a true additional risk factor.

REFERENCES

1 Stokes PL, Asquith P, Holmes GTH, Mackintosh P and Cooke WT. Inheritance and influence of histocompatibility (HLA) antigens in adult coeliac disease. Gut 1973;14:627-730.

2 Tiwari J, Terasaki P. HLA and Disease Associations. Springer 1985;236-242.

3 Tosi R, Vismara D, Tanigaki N, Ferrara GB, Cicimarra F, Boffalano W, Follo D, Aurichio S. Evidence that coeliac disease is primarily associated with DC locus allelic specificity. Chri. Immunol Immunopath 1983;28:395-404.

4 Roep BO, Bontrop RE, Peña AS, van Eggermond MCJA, van Rood JJ, Giphart MJ. An HLA-DQ alpha allele identified at DNA and protein level is strongly associated with coeliac disease. Human Immunol 1988;23:271-9.

5 Sollid LM, Markussen G, Ek J, Gjerde H, Vartdal F, Thosby E. Evidence for a primary association of coeliac disease to a particular HLA-DQ α/β heterodimer. J Exp Med 1989;169:345-50.

6 Morellini M, Trabaces S, Mazzilli MC, Lulli P, Capellacci S, Bonamico M, Margarit I, Gandidi E. A study of HLA class II antigens in an Italian paediatric population with coeliac disease. Disease Markers 1988;6:23-28.

7 Bugawan T, Horn GT, Long CM, Mickelson E, Hansen JA, Ferrara GB, Angelini G, Erlich HA. Analysis of HLA-DP allelic sequence polymorphism using in vitro enzymatic DNA amplification of DP alpha and DP be Loci. J Immunol 1988;141:4024-4030.

8 Alper CA, Fleischnick E, Awdeh Z, Katz AJ and Yunis EJ. Extended major histocompatibility complex haplotypes in patients with gluten-sensitive enteropathy. J Clin 1987;79:251-256.

9 Hall MA, Lanchburry JSS, Bolsover WJ, Welch KI, Ciclitira PJ. Coeliac disease is associated with an extended HLA-DR3 haplotype which includes HLA-DPw1. Human Immunol 1989;27:220-228.

10 Rosenberg WML, Wordsworth BP, Jewell DP, Bell JI. A locus telomeric to HLA-DP encodes susceptibility to coeliac disease. Immonogenetics 1989;30:307-310.

11 Lundin KEA, Sollid LM, Qvigstad E, Markussen G, Gjertsen HA, Thorsby E. T lymphocyte recognition of a coeliac disease-associated cis or trans-encosed HLA-DQ α/β heterodimer. J Immunol 1990;145:136-139.

ADENOVIRUS 12 AND COELIAC DISEASE.

G.J. Mantzaris, M.D. and D.P. Jewell, D.Phil., FRCP. Gastroenterology Unit, Radcliffe Infirmary, Oxford, OX2 6HE, UK.

Well-documented cases of discordance for coeliac disease (CD) in monozygotic twins have raised the question whether environmental factors other than gluten are implicated in the pathogenesis of this disease. Exploring this possibility, Kagnoff et al. reported a striking similarity between the E1b protein of the human intestinal adenovirus 12 (Ad12) and A-gliadin, a toxic polymer of α-gliadins. The region of homology includes 8 identities over a span of 12 amino acids. Kagnoff et al. postulated that by virtue of immunological cross-reactivity an infection with Ad12 might render a genetically susceptible individual liable to become sensitized to gluten in such a way as to lead on to small intestinal damage. In support of this, coeliac patients have raised titres of neutralizing antibodies to Ad12, but not to adenovirus 18 and ECHO-virus 11. However, antibodies to the E1b protein could not be demonstrated. Despite these conflicting results on aspects of the humoral immunity to Ad12, lymphocytes of treated coeliac patients in remission, but not those of healthy subjects and patients with inflammatory bowel disease, elicited marked and dose-dependent immune responses when challenged with synthetic dodecapeptides from the viral and the gliadin epitopes in leucocyte migration inhibition assays and proliferation assays. There was also a highly significant correlation between response obtained with both viral and gliadin peptides. Furthermore, a cyanogen bromide fragment of A-gliadin, which contains the gliadin dodecapeptide, showed toxicity for untreated coeliac jejunal mucosa in organ culture. Nevertheless, since the demonstration of a cellular immune response to these peptides does not indicate that they are toxic <u>in vivo</u>, we have instilled 100 mg of the gliadin synthetic dodecapeptide into the duodenum of two treated coeliac patients and two non-coeliac patients. Biopsies were taken before and over the subsequent 24 hours following the instillation of the peptide. We found that significant biochemical, histological and cellular changes occured in the coeliac, but not in the control individuals. It is possible that there are peptides within α-gliadin molecule other than the dodecapeptide which can also mediate a toxic response. There also may be several such peptides which may or may not cross-react with peptides in other infective organisms. However, at the present time it is reasonable to consider that a pathogen, be that Ad12 or another pathogen, cross-reacting with the gliadin molecule may trigger the onset of CD in genetically susceptible individuals.

INTRODUCTION

CD develops in genetically susceptible individuals who consume gluten and treatment is achieved by means of a gluten-free diet (GFD). However, studies have documented the lack of complete concordance for the disease in monozygotic twins and HLA indentical siblings (1), as well as the failure of excess gluten intake to induce small intestinal damage in unaffected subjects of these groups (2). Variations have also been documented in the incidence of CD in recent years (3). These obser-

M. L. Mearin and C. J. J. Mulder (eds.), Coeliac Disease, 15–19.

vations have raised the question whether enviromental factors other than gluten are implicated in the pathogenesis of this disease.

ADENOVIRUS 12

Exploring this hypothesis, Kagnoff reported a striking resemblance in the amino-acid sequences of the E1b protein from the human adenovirus 12 (Ad12) and A-gliadin (4). A-gliadin is a toxic polymer of α-gliadins whose primary structure is known: it consists of 266 amino-acids arranged in five domains (5). Adenoviruses cause gastrointestinal infections in humans as early as the first year of life, which are usually asymptomatic (6). Ad12 is not amongst the commonest adenoviruses, but is has been thoroughly studied because of its ability to transform mammalian cell lines (7). The latter is probably due to a reduced expression of MHC Class I antigens on the surface of infected cells. The E1b protein is encoded for by the genomic region which is responsible for the transforming ability of Ad12. It is released in the cytoplasm of the transformed cells during the early stages of the lytic infection and is not a structural protein (7). The region of sequence homology spans 12 amino-acids (residues 206-217 in A-gliadin and 384-395 in Ad12E1b protein) and includes 8 identities (Fig I). These sequences are hydrophilic and are therefore likely to be located on the surface of the two molecules (4). Kagnoff postulated that by virtue of immunological cross-reactivity between these shared epitopes an infection with Ad12 might render a genetically susceptible individual to become liable to gluten sensitization in such a way as to lead on to CD. In support of this, they reported that antisera raised to Ad12 cross-react with whole gliadin, a cyanogen-bromide fragment of A-gliadin (residues 128-246, which contained the gliadin dodecapeptide) and a heptapeptide from within the region of sequence homology (4). Further evidence has come from a study of neutralizing antibodies to Ad12 and other intestinal viruses: coeliac patients showed evidence of prior infection with Ad12 but not with a closely related adenovirus, Ad18, or echovirus 11. In contrast, neutralizing antibodies to Ad12 were rarely found in healthy subjects and patients with other intestinal diseases (8). However, doubts have been cast on this hypothesis by Howdle, who could not demonstrate antibodies to the Ad12E1b protein by radioimmunoprecipitation (9). We and others have reported contradictory results regarding the presence of antibodies to the A-gliadin dodecapeptide in the serum of coeliac patients (9-11).

FIGURE I REGION OF SEQUENCE HOMOLOGY IN THE MOLECULES OF A-GLIADIN AND THE Ad12Elb PROTEIN.

A-gliadin (206-217)
Leu-Gly-Gln-Gly-Ser-Phe-Arg-Pro-Ser-Gln-Gln-Asn

Leu-Arg-Arg-Gly-Met-Phe-Arg-Pro-Ser-Gln-Cys-Asn
Ad12E1b protein (384-395)

CELLULAR HYPERSENSITIVITY

In Oxford, we have studied the cellular immune responses of coeliac patients and control subjects to synthetic dodecapeptides from the viral and the gliadin epitopes. These peptides were synthesized by solid phase methods and, after purification, were shown to run as a single peak in reverse-phase HPLC. Using an indirect leucocyte migration inhibition assay (LMIA), we initially showed that peripheral blood mononuclear cells (PB MNC) of treated coeliac patients in remission on a GFD elicited marked, dose-dependent immune responses when challenged with three different concentrations of the gliadin synthetic peptide (12). The majority of healthy control subjects and patients with inflammatory bowel disease did not demonstrate such responses. Cells of patients with untreated coeliac disease also did not react to the gliadin peptide, but immune responsiveness was detected once these patients went into remission on a strict GFD. Presumably, the sensitized cells are predominantly in the inflamed intestinal mucosa in the untreated condition, but following gluten withdrawal from the diet they depart the intestine and can easily be detected in the peripheral blood. Subsequently, we have shown that a synthetic dodecapeptide from the viral epitope will also stimulate PB MNC of treated coeliac patients, but not those of healthy and disease controls. The cellular immune response to the viral peptide is closely correlated with the response to the gliadin peptide using either LMIA or proliferation assays (13). Although in these experiments PB MNC were used, the results reflect T cell sensitization to these peptides for two reasons. Firstly, PM MNC of treated coeliac patients were shown to release a substance with many of the properties of leucocyte migration inhibition factor following challenge with the gliadin synthetic peptide (14). Secondly, a significant correlation was found between migration indices obtained from treated coeliac patients using unfractionated PB MNC and a highly purified PB T cell population (16). Therefore, the observed immune responses are most probably due to the release of migration inhibition factor by sensitized T lymphocytes, and consequently, they truly reflect cellular hypersensitivity to the gliadin and the viral epitopes. This was further supported by the observation that the proliferative responses of PB MNC of treated coeliac patients, but not of healthy subjects, to both gliadin and viral synthetic peptides were also marked, dose-dependent and significantly correlated with each other. These in vitro immune responses were not influenced by a particular HLA haplotype, since neither coeliac patients nor control individuals, who had identical HLA haplotypes, showed similar hypersensitivity. In addition, no single HLA haplotype could be identified within the coeliac group which determined a marked immune response, although coeliac patients who had HLA B8 DR3 DQ2 tended to be stronger responders (12,15).

CHALLENGE STUDIES

Immunological hypersensitivity for an antigen does not necessarily imply a pathogenetic role for that antigen and for CD feeding studies are essential to determine toxicity. These have now been performed using the synthetic gliadin peptide. 100 mg peptide dissolved in 50 ml normal saline were instilled into the duodenum of two treated coeliac patients in remission on a GFD and two patients who were being investigated for symptoms of irritable bowel symdrome. In serial biopsy specimens over the subsequent 24 hours, significant biochemical, histological and cellular changes were seen in the coeliac but not in the control group. Thus, the synthetic gliadin peptide appears to be toxic (16). It is reasonable to assume that this toxic effect was due to the activation of immunological effector mechanisms, since the A-gliadin sequence is hydrophilic (4), binds avidly to DR3 molecules expressed on the surface of EBV-transformed B lymphocytes (Dr J Rothbard, Personal Communication), and elicits cellular immune responses in vitro. However, it does not necessarily follow that this particular epitope is the only epitope in gliadin that mediates toxicity.

DISCUSSION

The possibility that a viral infection may trigger CD in genetically susceptible individuals by virtue of a chance immunological cross-reactivity with gliadin at the level of the T cell receptor is not only intriguing but may also explain some of the epidemiological aspects of this disease. According to this hypothesis, an MHC-immune response gene, which underlies CD, is activated by an infection with Ad12. This initiates an inappropriate immune response which is then subsequently perpetuated by the ingestion of gliadin. However, other mechanisms have also been considered. In this respect, Carter (17) examined the possibility that Ad12 might establish a chronic intestinal infection leading to small intestinal damage, but they were unable to identify viral DNA in duodenal biopsies from coeliac patients using Southern blot techniques (17). However, this does not exclude the possibility that a persistent Ad12 infection may form a link between CD and its major complication, intestinal lymphoma, given the transforming ability of Ad12. Our results as well as those of Kagnoff (4) favour the former hypothesis, but do not prove it. Coeliac patients may be more vulnerable to infections with Ad12 possibly because of abnormalities of the intestinal epithelium and, therefore, the evidence of a prior Ad12 infection may not be directly related to the pathogenesis of CD. Furthermore, many questions need to be answered. We do not know whether the A-gliadin (206-217) sequence is the only peptide within α-gliadin molecule which can mediate a toxic response. There is some evidence that A-gliadin derived peptides containing two tetrapeptide sequences, namely Pro-Ser-Gln-Gln and Gln-Gln-Gln-Pro, can mediate a toxic effect for unteated coeliac jejunal mucosa in organ culture assays (18). Although the role of these tetrapeptides in CD is virtually unknown, they may well be part of the toxic epitope(s). The former of these tetrapeptides is contained in the gliadin dodecapeptide and has been found in alpha-type gliadins for which sequences have been reported, but not in other types of wheat storage proteins of known primary structure. However, Kagnoff (4) have reported that the gliadin dodecapeptide sequence was demonstrated in other alpha- and beta-gliadins by Western immunoblotting. On the other hand, there may be several such peptides in gliadins which may cross-react with amino-acid sequences in other infective organisms. Finally, factors other than environmental pathogens may also be responsible for discordance amongst HLA identical individuals. One such factor could be variability of gene rearrangement which is known to occur in the generation of T cell receptors. This diversity could be expected to result in differences in T cell responses even in genetically identical individuals (19). However, at the present time it is reasonable to consider that the onset of CD may be triggered in a genetically susceptible individual if he/she is exposed to an infection such as Ad12 which can cross-react with gliadin.

REFERENCES

1 Polanco I, Biemond I, Van Leeuwen A, et al. Gluten-sensitive enteropathy in Spain: genetic and environmental factors. In; McConnell RB, ed. The genetics of coeliac disease. Lancaster, England, MTP Press, 1981: 211-31.
2 Polanco I, Mearin ML, Larrauri J, Biemond I, Wipkink-Bakker A, Peña AS. Effect of gluten supplementation in healthy siblings of children with coeliac disease. Gastroenterology 1987; 92: 678-81.
3 Midhagen G, Jarnerot G, Kraaz W. Adult coeliac disease within a defined geographic area in Sweden. Scand J Gastroenterology 1988; 23:1000-1004.
4 Kagnoff MF, Austin RK, Hubert JJ, Kasarda DD. Possible role for a human adenovirus in the pathogenesis of coeliac disease. J Exp Med 1984; 160:1544-57.
5 Kasarda DD, Okita TW, Bernadin JE, et al. Nucleic acid (cDNA) and amino acid sequences of a-type gliadin of wheat (Tricitum aevistum L). Proc Natl Acad Sci USA 1984; 81:4712-6.
6 Willcocks MM, Carter MJ, Laidler F, Madeley CR. Restriction enzyme analysis of faecal adenovirus in Newcastle-upon-Tyne. Epidemiol Infect 1988; 101:445-58.
7 Kirmura T, Sawada Y, Shinawawa M, et al. Nucleotide sequence of the transforming early region E1b of adenovirus type 12 DNA: structure and gene organization, and comparison with those of adenovirus 5 DNA. Nucleic Acid Res 1981; 9:6571-89.
8 Kagnoff MF, Paterson YJ, Kumar PJ, Kasarda DD, Carbone FR. Unsworth DJ, Austin RK. Evidence for a role of a human intestinal adenovirus in the pathogenesis of coeliac disease. Gut 1987; 28:995-1001.
9 Howdle PD, Blair Zajdel ME, Smart CJ, Trejdosiewicz LK, Blair GE, Losowsky MS. Lack of a serologic response to an E1b protein of adenovirus 12 in coeliac disease. Scand J Gastroenterology 1989; 24:282-6.
10 Devery JM, La Brooy JT, Krillis S, Davidson G, Skerrit JH. Antigliadin antibody specificity for gluten-derived peptides toxic to coeliac patients. Clin Exp Immunol 1989; 76:384-90.
11 Nanda R, Carrington J, Priddle JD, Jewell DP. Serum antibodies to gliadin and a synthetic dodecapeptide from gliadin in coeliac disease. Submitted for publication.
12 Karagiannis JA, Priddle JD, Jewell DP. Cell-mediated immunity to a synthetic gliadin peptide resembling a sequence from adenovirus 12. Lancet 1987; i:884-6.
13 Mantzaris GJ, Karagiannis JA, Priddle JD, Jewell DP. Cellular hypersensitivity to a synthetic dodecapeptide derived from the adenovirus 12 which resembles a sequence of α-gliadin in patients with coeliac disease. Gut 1990; 31:668-73.
14 Lydford-Davies H, Karagiannis JA, Priddle JD, Jewell DP. Preliminary characterization of leucocyte migration inhibition factor (LIF) produced by lymphocytes from coeliac patients when stimulated with gluten peptides. Clin Sci 1987; 72 (suppl): 89.
15 Mantzaris GJ, Priddle JD, Jewell DP. T lymphocyte responses to a dodecapeptide from adenovirus 12 in coeliac patients. J Clin Lab Immunol 1990; in press.
16 Mantzaris GJ, Jewell DP. In vivo toxicity of a synthetic dodecapeptide from A gliadin in patients with coeliac disease. Scand J Gastroenterol: in press.
17 Carter MJ, Willcocks MM, Mitchison HC, Record CO, Madeley CR. Is a persistent adenovirus infection involved in the pathogenesis of coeliac disease? Gut 1989; 30:1563-7.
18 De Ritis G, Auricchio S, Jones HW, Lew EJ-L, Bernadin JE, Kasarda DD. In vitro (organ culture) studies of the toxicity of specific A-gliadin peptides in coeliac disease. Gastroenterology 1988; 94:41-9.
19 Rosenberg W, Jewell DP, Bell IL. In preparation.

GLIADIN PEPTIDES: THEIR EFFECT ON THE GUT MUCOSA.

S. Auricchio, R. Troncone, Dep.Pediatrics, University of Naples, via S. Pansini 5, I-80131, Naples, Italy.

The effect of gliadin peptides on the gut mucosa has been investigated both by in vivo (jejunal and rectal challenges) and in vitro studies. This paper will deal with in vitro studies, aimed to identify the toxic proteins and peptides, to study the mechanisms of mucosal damage, and to assess the possibility of protecting the coeliac intestine from their toxic activity. The organ culture of small intestine from untreated patients has been proposed as an in vitro model of coeliac disease (CD). No improvement, but damage occurs when jejunum from untreated patients is cultured in the presence of gliadin peptides. Other methods have also been developed which probably reveal a non-immunomediated cytotoxic activity of gliadin peptides on the small intestine and other cells. In fact, gliadin peptides reversibly inhibit development and morphogenesis of the very inmature small intestine of a 17-day old fetus; they are also able to agglutinate human K562 (S) cells, a line of chronic myeloid leukemia. The proteins and peptides that in vitro and/or in vivo are toxic for the coeliac small intestine are also able to damage the in vitro developing fetal rat intestine and to agglutinate K562 (S) cells. It is likely that the unknown mechanism(s) underlying these latter two activities of some gliadin peptides may be involved in the pathogenesis of the intestinal lesion in CD. These in vitro methods have been used to identify the toxic proteins and peptides. Experiments performed testing A-gliadin peptides of known amino acid sequence have shown that the gliadin toxicity resides in the N-terminal portion of the molecule, and that the largest sequences common to toxic peptides are pro-ser-gln-gln and gln-gln-gln-pro, these sequences being absent from non-toxic peptides. These in vitro models have also been extensively used to study the mechanisms of the damaging activity of gliadin peptides on the coeliac intestine. More recently, subtle changes have become apparent in jejunal specimens from patients in remission, cultured in the presence of gliadin peptides. The biosynthesis of some brush border hydrolases has been demonstrated to be severely decreased; furthermore, gliadin peptides are able to change the distribution of class II molecules on the epithelial cells, inducing the expression of HLA-DR antigens in the crypts and their disappearance from the surface of the villous cells. Finally, these in vitro methods enable the study of new possible dietetic or pharmacologic therapy of the disease. In fact, they can be used for screening wheat varieties in search of wheats which could be non-toxic for coeliac patients. They can also be used to test ways of making gliadins non-toxic for the coeliac mucosa, and to detect compounds able to protect coeliac mucosa from the damaging effect of gliadin peptides.

INTRODUCTION

The effect of gliadin peptides on the gut mucosa has been investigated both by in vivo (jejunal and rectal challenges) and in vitro studies. This paper will deal with in vitro studies aimed to identify the toxic proteins and peptides, to study the mechanisms of mucosal damage, and to assess the possibility of protecting the coeliac intestine from their toxic activity.

M. L. Mearin and C. J. J. Mulder (eds.), Coeliac Disease, 21–26.

IN VITRO METHODS FOR THE STUDY OF COELIAC DISEASE

The organ culture of human small intestine has been proposed as an in vitro model of CD (1,2). Jejunal specimens obtained from patients with active enteropathy show morphologic and biochemical improvement when cultured in a medium free from gliadin peptides. No improvement, but damage occurs when the tissue is cultured in the presence of gliadin peptides (1-4). These observations have been found to be specific to prolamines toxic for CD patients, but not specific to coeliac atrophy (5). On the contrary, the mucosal architecture of the histologically normal jejunum from coeliac patients on a gluten-free diet has been found not to be affected by the presence of gliadin in the culture medium. More recently, the organ culture of jejunum from coeliac patients in remission has been reappraised as an investigative tool of mucosal immunity. In fact, gliadin peptides do induce HLA-DR expression in the crypt epithelium of cultured mucosa (6). This phenomenon is likely to be the result of cytokine production, following the activation of gliadin specific T cells in the jejunal mucosa. As currently there are no standard methods for detecting the presence of antigen specific cells in the mucosa, these observations propose a new in vitro model which could prove useful for the identification of the gliadin epitopes involved in the activation of the specific mucosal cell-mediated immune response. The other observation made in the great majority of biopsy specimens from coeliac subjects, cultured in the presence of gliadin peptides, is the disappearance of HLA DR molecules from the villous mucosal surface during the organ culture. The mechanism underlying this phenomenon is more difficult to interpret, but our data are on the same line as other recent observations. In fact, the biosynthesis of some brush border hydrolases has been demonstrated to be severely decreased by culturing the histologically normal coeliac intestine in the presence of gliadin peptides (7). It is possible that gliadin interferes with the protein syntesis machinery of the coeliac intestine epithelial cell, and/or with the transport of glycoproteins to the brush border.
Other methods have been developed for the study of cereal components toxic in CD, which probably reveal a non-immunomediated cytotoxic activity of gliadin peptides on the small intestine and other cells. Gliadin peptides reversibly inhibit development and morphogenesis of the very immature small intestine of a 17-day old rat fetus, whereas they have no effect on the in vitro cultured differentiated jejunum from a 21-day old rat fetus; this observation shows that gliadin peptides may have a direct damaging activity against the small intestinal mucosa only during an early phase of its morphogenesis (8-10). Similar results have been obtained by culturing the fetal chick intestine in the presence of gliadin peptides, and monitoring the increase of disaccharidase activity as a measure of intestinal differentiation (11).
A further biological activity of gliadin peptides probably, related to their toxicity for CD patients, is their ability to agglutinate human K562 (S) cells, a line of chronic myeloid leukemia (12). The proteins and peptides that in vivo and/or in vitro are toxic for the coeliac small intestine (bread wheat gliadins and gliadin peptides; prolamines and prolamine peptides from rye, oats, and barley; some A gliadin peptides) are able to damage the in vitro developing fetal rat intestine and to agglutinate, at very low concentration, K 562 (S) cells. The peptides that in vivo and/or in vitro are non toxic for coeliacs (bread wheat albumin, globulin and glutenin peptides; durum wheat gliadin peptides; prolamin peptides from rice and maize; some other A-gliadin peptides) are unable to damage the in vitro developing fetal rat

intestine and to agglutinate K cells (8-10,12,13). Therefore, the toxic activity in vivo and in vitro for the coeliac intestine of a large series of proteins, mixtures of peptides, and pure A-gliadin peptides correlates very well with the cell agglutinating activity and the damaging effect on the in vitro developing fetal rat intestine. This suggests that the unknown mechanism(s) underlying these latter two activities of some gliadin peptides may be involved in the pathogenesis of the intestinal lesion in CD.

TOXIC PROTEINS AND PEPTIDES

During the last years, these three in vitro methods have been used to identify the toxic proteins and peptides. The α-gliadin class of gliadins is toxic when included in the culture medium of flat coeliac mucosa (1,14,15). In vitro (15,16) studies have demonstrated that not only α-gliadin, but also β, Γ and Ω gliadins and genetic variants of hexaploid wheats with low α-gliadin content (17,18) are toxic. Although in vitro experiments suggest that durum wheat gliadin peptides are less toxic than bread wheat gliadin peptides (8), preliminary in vivo studies (Auricchio, unpublished observations) indicate that durum wheat also causes atrophy of the coeliac duodenal mucosa. Therefore, the damaging effect on the coeliac intestine is apparently a property common to different wheat varieties and gliadin classes, although more extensive studies should be done before a definite conclusion can be drawn. Most interestingly, such models, particularly the organ culture of untreated coeliac mucosa, have been used to identify putative toxic sequence(s) of gliadin. Several A-gliadin derived peptides have been tested for their toxicity on in vitro cultured, untreated coeliac mucosa. Three peptides derived by cyanogen bromide cleavage (CN I, II and III) span the complete aminoacid sequence of A-gliadin, which is made of 266 aminoacid residues. The first two fragments are toxic, whereas the third fragment is non-toxic. The CN I residue, formed by the first 127 aminoacids is split by chymotrypsin in various fragments. The fragment XT1 corresponding to the first 55 aminoacids and its two parts XT 1-30 and XT 31-55 are all toxic, whereas the peptide XT 56-68 is non toxic. The largest aminoacid sequences which are common to the toxic peptides and absent in the non toxic peptides are pro-ser-gln-gln and gln-gln-gln-pro (19). Comparable results have been obtained by Weiser (20,21).

MECHANISMS OF DAMAGE

These in vitro models have also been extensively used to study the mechanisms of the damaging activity of gliadin peptides on the coeliac intestine. The observation that the damaging effect of gliadin peptides on in vitro cultured flat coeliac mucosa is abolished by corticosteroids, has been used to implicate immunologic mechanisms in the causation of mucosal damage (22). Furthermore, jejunal mucosa specimens from coeliac patients in remission are not affected (or much less affected) than biopsies from untreated patients by the presence of gliadin in culture medium. In vivo challenge with gluten makes the small intestine of patients in remission sensitive to the in vitro damaging effect of gliadin peptides. Furthermore, coeliac mucosa in remission when co-cultured with flat coeliac mucosa (23), or with lymphocytes from blood of coeliacs (24), is damaged in vitro by gliadin peptides. Finally, as already mentioned, gliadin peptides do induce HLA-DR expression in the crypt epithelium of cultured mucosa from patients in remission (6). It has, therefore, been suggested that in patients in remission gliadin must first initiate a set of immunological events in vivo, before the cytotoxic effect on enterocytes can be displayed in vitro. On the other hand, a direct, non immunomediated cytotoxic activity of gliadin peptides on the small intestine may also be involved in the pathogenesis of CD, as suggested by the previously reported studies showing that gliadin and prolamines peptides, toxic both in vitro and in vivo, cause reversible inhibition of the in vitro development of the fetal rat intestine and agglutinate undifferentiated human K 562 (S) cells.

PROTECTIVE MECHANISMS

Finally, these in vitro methods enable the study of new possible dietetic or pharmacologic therapy of the disease (12,13,25-27). In fact, they could be used for screening wheat varieties in search of wheats which could be non toxic for CD patients. Furthermore, they could be used to test ways of making gliadins non toxic for the coeliac mucosa. They could also be used to detect compounds able to protect coeliac mucosa from the damaging effect of gliadin peptides. Mannan and oligomers of N-acetylglucosamine, N,N'-diacetylchitobiose and N,N',N"-triacetylchitotriose are able to prevent the cell agglutinating activity and the damaging in vitro effect, both on the developing fetal rat intestine, and on the flat coeliac mucosa of the active peptides (12,13,25,26). Furthermore, mannan specifically binds only a few peptides of a gliadin digest, which are the only ones active in damaging in vitro the fetal rat intestine and in agglutinating K 562 (S) cells (27). Studies based on the hypothesis that amines may protect the coeliac small intestine from the damaging activity of gliadin peptides are currently being performed in vitro. They are suggested by the hypothesis that small intestinal transglutaminase could be involved in the mucosal handling of gliadins. Transglutaminases are Ca2+ -dependent enzymes crosslinking τ-carboxamide groups of peptide-bound glutamine residues and ϵ-aminogroups for peptide-bound lysine (28,29,30). Gliadins are very good and versatile substrate of transglutaminase (31). The intestinal transglutaminase activity present on the mucosal surface, or released in the lumen, is involved in vitro in the metabolism of gliadins and their peptides, possibly crosslinking these proteins to cell membrane (Auricchio, unpublished results). Whether such processes have anything to do with the mucosal handling of gliadin in relationship to CD is still a matter of speculation. As a matter of fact, various amines, among which the most active are spermidine, spermine and putrescine, are able to inhibit the agglutinating activity of gliadin peptides. Spermidine is also able to protect the in vitro developing fetal rat intestine, and the atrophic coeliac intestine, from the toxic activity of gliadin peptides (32). It is possible to speculate that these effects might be related to an interference by amines on the process of gliadin binding and endocytosis.

CONCLUSIONS

It is likely that immunologic mechanisms play a major role in causing the small intestinal lesions of CD. Nevertheless, whether the primary disturbance is immunologic in nature, or rather metabolic, is still a matter of debate. The primary immune defect theory (33) is in principle not in contrast with the other damaging mechanisms of gliadin peptides discussed in this paper. The direct cytotoxic activity of gliadin peptides and/or their abnormal mucosal handling could be in fact related to the targetting of the small intestinal mucosa for the immunologic reactions against gliadin.

REFERENCES

1 Falchuk ZM, Gebhard RL, Sessoms C, Strober W. An in vitro model of gluten-sensitive enteropathy. J Clin Invest 1974;53:487.
2 Jos J, Lenoir G, de Ritis G, Rey J. In vitro pathogenetic studies of coeliac intestinal biopsy specimens maintained in culture for 48 hours. Scand J Gastroenterol 1975;10:121.
3 Fluge G, Askens L. Labelling indices after 3H-thymidine incorporation during organ culture of duodenal mucosa in coeliac disease. Scand J Gastroenterol 1981;16:921.
4 Howdle PD, Corazza GR, Bullen AW, Losowski MS. In vitro demonstration of mucosal sensivity to gluten. Gut 1979;20:436.
5 Olives JP, Schmitz J, Jos J, Detand MF, Rey J. In vitro intestinal citotoxicity of various fractions from gliadin and cows milk protein in children. Quantitative assessment by a morphometric method. Gastroenterol Clin Biol 1982;6:557.
6 Fais S. Maiuri L, Troncone R, de Ritis G, Pallone F, Auricchio S. Gliadin induces HLA DR expression on crypt epithelium during organ culture of treated coeliac mucosa. International Congress of Mucosal Immunology, London, 24-26 July 1989.
7 Naim HY, Ambhul P, Sterchi EE, Gaze H, Lentze MJ. An in vitro model system for studying the biosynthesis of brush border membrane (BBM) hydrolases in coeliac disease. Pediatr Res 1987;22:102.
8 Auricchio S, de Ritis G, De Vincenzi M, Occorsio P, Silano V. Effect of gliadin peptides prepared from hexaploid and tetraploid wheat on cultures of intestine from rat fetuses and celiac children. Pediatr Res 1982;16:1004.
9 Auricchio S, Cardelli M, de Ritis G, De Vincenzi M, Latte F, Silano V. An in vitro animal model for the study of cereal components toxic in celiac disease. Pediatr Res 1984;18:1372.
10 de Ritis G, Occorsio P, Auricchio S, Gramenzi F, Morisi G, Silano V. Toxicity of wheat flour proteins and protein-derived peptides for in vitro developing intestine from rat fetus. Pediatr Res 1979;13:1255.
11 Mothes TH. International Symposium on Brush Border Membranes. Bern 4-7 November, 1987.
12 Auricchio S, de Ritis G, De Vincenzi M, Mancini M, Minetti M, Sapora O, Silano V. Agglutinating activity of gliadin-derived peptides from bread wheat: Implications for celiac disease pathogenesis. Biochem Biophys Res Comm 1982;121:428.
13 Auricchio S, de Ritis G, De Vincenzi M, Silano V. Toxicity mechanisms of wheat and other cereals in coeliac disease and related enteropathies. J Pediatr Gastroenterol Nutr 1985;4:923.
14 Falchuk ZM, Nelson DL, Katz AJ, Bernardin JE, Kasarda DD, Hague NE, Strober W. Gluten sensitive enteropathy: Influence of hystocompatibility type on gluten sensitivity in vitro. J Clin Invest 1980;66:227.
15 Jos J, Charbonnier L, Mosse J, Olives JP, de Tand MF, Rey J. The toxic fraction of gliadin digest in coeliac disease. Isolation by chromatography on Biogel-10. Clin Chim Acta 1982;119:263.
16 Howdle PD, Ciclitira PJ, Simpson FG, Losowsky MS. Are all gliadins toxic in celiac disease? An in vitro study of α,β,τ and w-gliadins. Scand J Gastroenterol 1984;19:41.
17 Ciclitira PJ, Hunter JO, Lennox ES. Clinical testing of bread made from mullisonic 6A wheat in coeliac patients. Lancet 1980;2:234.
18 Kasarda DD. Protein and peptides in coeliac disease: relation to cereal genetics. In: Walker DN, Kretchmer N, eds. Food Nutrition and Evolution. Masson Publishing, New York, 1981, p 201.
19 de Ritis G, Auricchio S, Holly WJ, Lew EJL, Bernardin JE, Kasarda DD. In vitro (organ culture) studies of the toxicity of specific A-gliadin peptides in celiac disease. Gastroenterology 1988;94;41.
20 Wieser H, Belitz HD, Ashkenazi A. Aminoacid sequence of the coeliac active peptide B 3142. Z Lebensm Unters Forsch 1984;179:371.
21 Wieser H, Belitz HD, Idar D, Ashkenazi A. Coeliac activity of the gliadin peptides CT-1 and CT-2. Z Lebensm Unter Forsch 1986;182:115.

22 Katz AJ, Falchuk ZM, Strober W, Scwachman H. In vitro study of the effect of cortisol. N Engl J Med 1976;295:131.
23 Falchuk ZM, Gebhard RL, Strober W. The pathogenesis of gluten-sensitive enteropathy (coeliac sprue): organ culture studies. In: Hekkens WTJM, Pena AS, eds. Coeliac disease. Proceedings of 2nd International Symposium. Stenfert Kroese, Leiden, 1974, p 107.
24 Simpson FG, Howdle PD, Robertson DAF, Losowsky MS. Jejunal biopsy and lymphocytes coculture in coeliac disease. Scand J Gastroenterol 1983;18:749.
25 Auricchio S, de Ritis G, De Vincenzi M, Occorsio P, Silano V. Prevention by mannan and other sugars of the in vitro damage of fetal rat intestine induced from cereals prolamine peptides toxic for human celiac intestine. Pediatr Res 1987;22:703.
26 de Ritis G, Auricchio S, De Vincenzi M, Mancini E, Minetti E, Sapora O, Silano V. Mannan prevents the in vitro toxicity of gliadin peptides (GP) on culture of coeliac mucosa and fetal rat intestine. Pediatr Res 1984;18:1052.
27 Maiuri L, Auricchio S, Cardelli M, de Ritis G, De Vincenzi M, Latte F, Mancini M, Raia V, Silano V. Selective binding to mannan of gliadin peptides which agglutinate undifferentiated K 562 cells and inhibit in vitro development of fetal rat intestine. Pediatr Res 1987;22:102.
28 Folk GE, Chung SI. Transglutaminases. Meth Enzimol 1985;113:358.
29 Lorand L, Conrad SM. Transglutaminases. Mol Cell Biochem 1984;58:9.
30 William-Hashman HG, Canellakis ZN. Transglutaminase-mediated covalent attachment of polyamines to protein: Mechanism and potential physiological significance. Physiol Chem Physic 1980;12:457.
31 Gentile V, Auricchio S, Porta R, Migliavacca M, Capano G, Auricchio S. Are soluble and/or membrane bound transglutaminase activities involved in intestinal metabolism of gliadins? Pediatr Res 1987;22:103.
32 Auricchio S, de Ritis G, De Vincenzi M, Gentile V, Maivci L, Mancini E, Porta R, Raia V. Amines protect in vitro the coeliac small intestine from the damaging activity of gliadin peptides. Gastroenterology (in press).
33 Strober W. An immunological theory of gluten sensitive enteropathy. In: Mc Nicholl B, McCarthy CF, Fottrell PF, eds. Perspectives in coeliac disease. MTP Press Limited, Lancaster, 1978, p 169.

HLA-DR-DP AND -DQ ANTIGENS IN COELIAC DISEASE

M. Luisa Mearin, Department of Paediatrics,
Leiden University Hospital, Box 9600, 2300 RC, Leiden, The Netherlands.

Population studies in different countries have confirmed the association of coeliac disease (CD) with the HLA class II molecules HLA-DR3 and -DR7, and with the HLA-DR phenotypes DR3/DR7, DR3/DR3 and DR5/DR7. Familystudies have also shown that CD segregates with these HLA-DR phenotypes. Among HLA-DR3-DR7 positive coeliac patients a 100% association of the disease with the HLA-class II molecule DQw2 has been described. Other reports have indicated an association between CD and some DP polymorphisms. Whether all those genes contribute to the susceptibility for CD or whether their association is secondary to the one with DQ is not known. One of the respects in which HLA-DQ molecules differ from HLA-DR ones is that both the α and the β chain genes are polymorphic in the HLA-DQ while polymorphism of the HLA-DR molecules is limited to the β chains. This is the reason why hybrid HLA-DQ molecules can result from genetranscomplementation. The HLA-DQw2 specificity is associated with two types of α/β dimers: DQ α 2.3/β 1.2 and with DQ α 2.7/β 2.7. On the other hand at DNA and at protein level it has been shown that CD is strongly associated with the HLA-DQ chains α 2.3, β 2.7 and β 2.3. It has been speculated that the HLA-DQ α 2.3/β 2.7 or the HLA-DQ α 2.3/β 2.3 dimers are the class II molecules involved in the onset of CD.
Because the mucosa of the small intestine of patients with CD is the target organ of the pathological mechanisms triggered by gliadin, the intestinal expression of the HLA class-II molecules associated to CD has been extensively investigated. Most studies have shown an increased expression of HLA-DR molecules both in epithelium and in the lamina propria lymphocytes of untreated CD patients. Significant stronger HLA-DP expression has been shown on the enterocytes of CD patients consuming gluten in comparison to CD patients on a gluten-free diet or to controls. Using specific monoclonal antibodies to the HLA-DQ α 2.3 and DQ β 2.7 chains our group has found that those chains are expressed in the lamina propria of the small intestine in both CD patients and HLA-matched controls. No expression was found on the enterocytes. One possible role for the class II molecules in the small intestinal epithelium of CD patients is that they may act as binding antigen molecules. If that is the case, it does not seem probable that the HLA-DQ heterodimers would be involved in the presentation of gliadin peptides. It is more likely that they may have a regulatory function in the immune response to gliadin.

INTRODUCTION

Susceptibility to CD is associated with genes that map to the class II D region of the HLA complex on chromosome 6 (1-7).
The HLA-complex genes are divided into 3 categories: class I, II and III and they encode the cell membrane antigens known as the HLA specificities (Figure 1). The HLA-complex genes class I and II have several subregions (class I: HLA-A, -B and -C; class II: HLA-DR-DQ, -DO, -DZ and -DP). Each subregion of the class II genes contains A and B genes which encode the α and β chains of the class II α/β heterodimers present on the cell surface (8). The combination of antigens encoded by

M. L. Mearin and C. J. J. Mulder (eds.), Coeliac Disease, 27–34.

one HLA chromosomal region is inherited as a unit: the HLA-haplotype. One of the characteristics of the HLA system is that some HLA-haplotype frequencies in the population are greater than would be expected from the products of the individual gene frequencies. Those allelic associations are named linkage disequilibrium and are often quite marked (e.g. HLA-A1-B8-DR3; HLA-A3-B7).

FIGURE I CHROMOSOME 6, MAJOR HISTOCOMPATIBILITY COMPLEX GENES AND THEIR PRODUCTS.

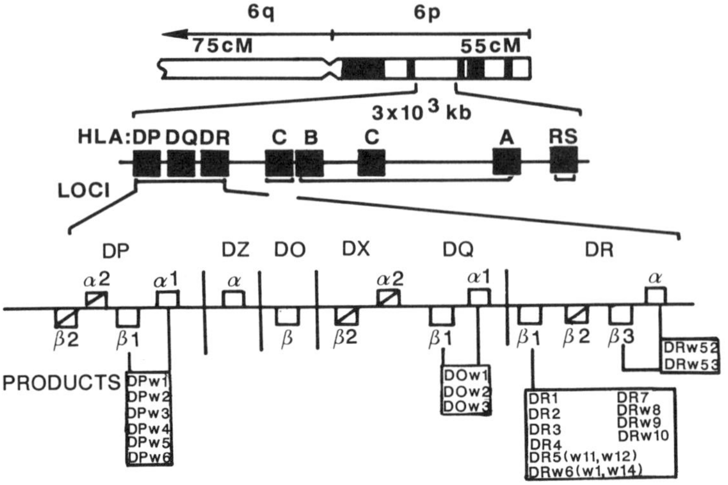

The first associations between CD and the HLA system were found with the class I molecules -A1 and -B8 (9,10), but later it was shown that CD was stronger associated with the HLA class II molecule -DW3 (1). The association with the class I molecules was found to be due to linkage disequilibrium. Population- and family studies have confirmed the association of CD with the HLA II molecules HLA-DR3 and -DR7 and with the HLA-DR phenotypes DR3/DR7, DR3/DR3 and DR5/DR7 (2,3; 11-14) (Table I).
In 1983 Tosi (4) described among HLA-DR3-DR7 positive coeliac patients, a 100% association of the disease with the HLA-class II molecule DQw2. Later investigations have shown that HLA-DR3-DR7 negative coeliac patients are not always HLA-DQw2 positive, but are DR4-positive (15). It has been noted too that the DR3 haplotype present among American black populations, which very unusually have CD, often lacks the DQw2 specificity (16).

TABLE I RELATIVE RISK OF SEVERAL HLA-DR PHENOTYPES FOR COELIAC DISEASE (CD)

HLA-DR PHENOTYPE	COUNTRY	YEAR	RELATIVE RISK (RR)
DR3/DR7	ITALY	1979	9.0
	FRANCE	1980	22.8
	ISRAEL	1981	15.1
	SPAIN	1983	11.5
	THE NETHERLANDS	1985	6.4
	ARGENTINA	1989	48.3
DR3/DR3	SPAIN	1983	21.8
	THE NETHERLANDS	1985	6.2
	ARGENTINA	1989	5.0
DR5/DR7	SPAIN	1983	3.7
	THE NETHERLANDS	1985	2.4
	ARGENTINA	1989	5.3

(RR = Risk of having CD when being positive for the HLA-DR phenotype in comparison with the risk for CD in the rest of the population)

One of the respects in which the HLA-DQ molecules differ from the HLA-DR ones, is that both the α and the β-chain genes are polymorphic in the HLA-DQ, polymorphism of the HLA-DR molecules is limited to the β-chains. This is the reason that hybrid HLA-DQ molecules can result from gene transcomplementation in heterozygous cells for DQ α and/or DQ β. Bontrop (17), using electrophoretic analysis of immunoprecipitated HLA-DQ molecules, could identify 10 different DQ α/β dimers within a panel of 29 HLA-DR-DQ homozygous B-cell lines. He found that the HLA-DQw2 allospecificity is associated with 2 types of α/β dimers: DQ $\alpha2.3/\beta2.3$ and with DQ $\alpha2.7/\beta2.7$. On the other hand, the same type of DQ α or DQ β chains can be expressed by cell lines with different HLA-DR-DQ haplotypes (Fig. 2). Thus it is possible, that the same HLA-DR α/β dimers are encoded by different HLA-DR-DQ haplotypes. In 1986 Howell (18) detected a 4.0 Kb RSA I fragment using a DQ β chain cDNA probe, among 9 from 10 CD patients and only in 1 from 5 DQw2-positive controls. In 1988 Roep (5) showed, at both the DNA and protein levels, that CD is strongly associated with the HLA-DQ chains $\alpha2.3$, $\beta2.7$ and to a lesser extent with the HLA-DQ $\beta2.3$ chain. From 2D gel analysis he concluded that at the cell surface HLA-DQ $\alpha2.3$ probably associates with the HLA-DQ $\beta2.7$ or HLA-DQ $\beta2.3$ chain. In some cases this association may be the result of transcomplementation; for example, the maternal haplotype may bring in the HLA-DQ $\alpha2.3$ whereas the paternal haplotype codes for the HLA-DQ $\beta2.7$. Recently Sollid (6) has shown that most of CD patients may share a particular HLA-DQ α/β heterodimer encoded by the combination of two HLA-DQ genes (HLA-DQA1 and DQB1). These genes are arranged in CIS position on the DR3DQw2 haplotype and in TRANS position in the DR5DQw7/DR7DQw2 heterozygous individuals.

FIGURE II THE SEROLOGICALLY DEFINED HLA-DQ ALLOSPECIFICI TIES -DQW1, -W2 AND -W3 CAN BE SPLITTED BASED UPON DQ ALPHA AND BETA CHAIN ISOELECTRIC POINTS (Bontrop 1987).

CELL LINE	HAPLOTYPE	DQ α pI-TYPE					DQ β pI - TYPE						
		1.1	1.2	1.12	2.3	2.7	1.1	1.2	1.12	1.19	2.3	2.7	3.4
OOS	DR1-Dw1-DQw1	■					■						
IWB	DR2-Dw2-DQw1		■					■					
SAS	DR2-Dw12-DQw1			■					■				
HHK	DRw13-Dw18-DQw1			■				■					
KRA	DRw13-Dw19-DQw1		■							■			
BRU	DRw14-Dw9-DQw1	■					■						
HAR	DR3-Dw3-DQw2				■						■		
EKR	DR7-Dw7-DQw2					■						■	
BSM	DR4-Dw4-DQw3				■			■					
MWM	DR4-Dw4-DQw3					■							■
ATH	DRw11-Dw5-DQw3				■								■
HLF	DRw12-DB6-DQw3				■								■
LUY	DRw8-Dw8-DQw3				■								■

His findings have greatly helped to understand why CD is associated with different HLA-DR-DQ haplotypes. It was already known by DNA analysis that the nucleotide sequences of the DR3DQw2 and DR5DQw7 haplotypes of the DQA1 genes and the DR3DQw2 and DR7DQw2 haplotypes of the DQB1 genes are almost identical (19), indicating a common origine of these genes. Thus, the genetic information of the DR3DQw2 haplotype is re-established in DR5DQw7/DR7DQw2 heterozygotes though the genes are split in two chromosomes.

Apart from the association between CD and the DR- and DQ-genes, other reports have indicated an association with some HLA-DP polymorphisms. However, the characterization of the DP molecules has in the past been limited by the lack of serology and the necessity to distinguish antigens using primed lymphocyte typing (PLT). By using this approach 6 different DP antigens were identified (20).
Niven (7) was the first to describe a relationship between CD and a 3.5 Kb fragment DP α gene digested by the BglII restriction enzyme (RR=6.8). No association with the serological markers DR or DQ was found and an independent association between CD and DP was postulated.
By restriction fragment length polymorphism (RFLP) analysis a 4.0 Kb RSaI DPB gene fragment was identified in more than in 90% of DR3(DRw17)DQw2 CD patients (21). Through molecular studies Bugawan (22) has found that the polymorphism of the DP molecules is much greater and larged confined to the β-chains. There are at least 21 DP specificities which can be detected using sequence-specific oligonucleotide (SSO) probes and polymerase chain reaction (PCR)-amplified

genomic DNA. Using this technique the distribution of the DP alleles in a group of Italian CD patients and controls has been studied and an increased frequency of DPB4.2 and DPB3 was found among the CD patients (23). The authors suggest that in different ethic groups different DP alleles may be associated with susceptibility to CD. Comparison of the DP sequences shows that the polymorphic residues at position 69, 56 and 57 which have been pointed as the putative peptide binding cleft and may therefore serve as peptides contact sites (24) may be critical in confering susceptibility. Further the contribution to the susceptibility for CD appeared to be independent of linkage disequilibrium with DR3 of DR7: the same proportion of DR3 and DR7 positive patients carried the DPB4.2 and DPB3 alleles.
However, using the same technique, Rosenberg (25) found that in an English Caucasian population only DP1 was significantly overrepresented among the CD patients and the DR3-controls. No increase in DPB4.2 or in DPB3 was detected in the CD group. All the DR3 patients and controls who had DPB1 possessed the full B8-DR3-DQw2 and DP1 haplotype suggesting a linkage disequilibrium of DPB1 with some B8-DR3 haplotype. The roughly equal subdivision between DPB1-positive and -negative B8-DR3 haplotypes in both CD patients and DR3 controls suggest that susceptibility genes are not likely to be in the portion of the haplotype that includes DP and must map in the MHC telomeric to the DP loci. Recently Herrera (14) analysed the frequency of certain HLA class II RFLP in 62 unrelated Argentinian CD patients and in 139 controls and found no significant overrepresentation of the DPB/RSaI 4.0 Kb fragment among the patients. The DPA/BgII 3.7 Kb fragment was neither increased among the CD population. Thus, the amount of evidence till now seems to point out an association of CD with an extended HLA-D haplotype in which the association with certain DP polymorphisms (DP1) is due to linkage disequilibrium with DR3DQw2.

THE HLA-II MOLECULES AND THE SMALL INTESTINE

The mucosa of the small intestine of patients with CD is the target organ of the pathological mechanism triggered by gliadin. According to the immunological theory for the etiology of CD it is tempting to speculate that the central defect resides in the abnormal immune response to gliadin mounted by the mucosa of the small intestine because of the presence of specific HLA class II molecules. Several studies on the subject have shown different patterns of HLA-class II molecules expressions at small intestine level in CD. Scott (26) was the first to report the expression of HLA-DR on normal villous epithelium in an apical granular distribution. More studies show increased expression of HLA-DR both in surface and crypt epithelium as well as in lamina propria lymphocytes of untreated CD patients (27-29). This increased epithelial class II expression is thought to be related to the immunological activity in the mucosa of CD patients. However, other groups have found opposite results i.e., a decrease of class II DR antigen expression in the enterocytes of untreated CD patients (30), even when the same technique was used (31). The significance of this findings remains unclear.
In their studies with frozen sections of jejunal mucosa from treated and untreated coeliac patients, Marley (29) found a pattern of DR<DP<DQ staining using monoclonal antibodies to the different class II antigenic specificities subgroups. The staining was observed most strongly in the villous enterocytes and decreased towards the crypt

bases. Kelly (32), in their studies on the differential expression of HLA-D gene products in the normal and coeliac small bowel using monoclonal antibodies, found that the HLA-DQ antigens showed a similar distribution, being absent from epithelial cells and present only in cells within the lamina propria.
Schweizer (33), using specific monoclonal antibodies to the HLA-DQ α2.3 and HLA-DQ β2.7 chains (which are highly associated to CD), has found that those chains are expressed in the lamina propria of the small intestine in both CD patients and HLA-matched controls. No expression of the HLA-DQ α2.3 or of the HLA-DQ β2.7 was found in the enterocytes of either group. Recently Bonamico (34), did not find HLA-DQ expression on the enterocytes of coeliac patients but dit show statistically significant differences in expression of DP antigens on enterocytes of coeliac patients on gluten containing diet or after gluten challenge in comparison with coeliac patients on a glutenfree diet or with controls. The HLA-DR, -DQ and -DP molecules are high polymorphic transmembrane proteins which bind peptides derived from the processing of foreign antigens and present them to the T-lymphocytes (35). They also influence the specificity of the mature T-cell repertoire (36). Most diseases showing association with HLA do associate with class II molecules. However, the underlying mechanisms which account for this relationship are not well understood. It is reasonable that the antigen-presenting capacity of a particular combination of class II molecules determines whether immunological response to a toxic substance is possible on a genetic level.
For CD, several models have been proposed, such as the HLA antigens serving as surface receptors for viruses or toxic substances, or the molecular mimicry of the HLA-molecules with the chemical structure of these substances allowing them to appear as self antigens (37). However, Gallagher (38) using fluorcitometry and EBV-transformed B-cell lines from coeliac patients and HLA-matched controls and mismatched controls could not show direct binding of α-gliadin to the HLA class II molecules of the B-cell lines nor could show a sharing of the antigenic determinant between α-gliadine and these molecules. At the small intestinal level two possible roles for class II molecules have been proposed (39). First, the enterocyte may be directly involved in antigen presentation. Second, enterocytes class II molecules may act as binding antigen molecules. If that is the case, it does not seem probable that the HLA-DQ heterodimers would be involved in the presentation of gliadin peptides in CD, but it is more likely that they have a regulatory function in the immune response once they have crossed the intestine epithelium. Whether the HLA-DR or -DP molecules may act as binding antigen molecules in CD deserves more investigation.

REFERENCES

1 Keuning JJ, Peña AS, van Leeuwen A, van Hoof JP, van Rood JJ. HLA-Dw3 associated with coeliac disease. Lancet 1976;i:506-7.
2 De Marchi M, Borelli Y, Olivetti E, Richardi P, Wright C, Ansaldi N, Barbera C, Santini B. Two HLA-D and DR alleles are associated with coeliac disease. Tissue Antigens 1979;14:309-16.
3 Mearin ML, Biemond I, Peña AS, Polanco I, Vazquez C, Schreuder GThM, de Vries RRP, van Rood JJ. HLA-DR phenotypes in Spanish coeliac children: their contribution to the understanding of the genetics of the disease. Gut 1983;24:532-7.
4 Tosi R, Vismara D, Tanigaki N, Ferrara GB, Cicimarra F, Boffalano W, Follo D, Aurichio S.

Evidence that celiac disease is primarily associated with a DC locus allelic specificity. Clin Immunol Immunopath 1983;28:395-404.
5 Roep BO, Bontrop RE, Peña AS, van Eggermond MCJA, van Rood JJ, Giphart MJ. An HLA-DQ alpha allele identified at DNA and protein level is strongly associated with coeliac disease. Human Immunol 1988;23:271-9.
6 Sollid LM, Markussen G, Ek J, Gjerde H, Vartdal F, Thorsby E. Evidence for a primary association of celiac disease to a particular HLA-DQ α/β heterodimer. J Exp Med 1989;169:345-50.
7 Niven MJ, Caffrey JC, Sachs JA, Cassell PG, Gallagher RB, Kumar P, Hitman GA. Susceptibility to coeliac disease involves genes in HLA-DP region. Lancet 1987;ii:805.
8 Korman AJ, Boss JM, Spies T, Sorrentino R, Okada K, Stominger JL. Genetic complexity and expression of human class II histocompatibility antigens. Immunol Rev 1985;85:45-86.
9 Stokes PL, Asquith P, Holmes GKT, MacKintosch P, Cooke WT. Histocompatibility antigens associated with adult coeliac disease. Lancet 1972;ii:162-4
10 Falchuck ZM, Rogentinc GN, Strober W. Predominance of histocompatibility antigen HLA8 in patients with gluten-sensitive enteropathy. J Clin Invest 1972;51:1602-5.
11 Betuel H, Gebuhrer L, Descos L, Percebois H, Minaire Y, Bertrand J. Adult celiac disease associated with HLA-DRw3 and -DRw7. Tissue Antigens 1980;15:231-42.
12 Brautbar C, Freier S, Ashkenazi A, Dekelbaum R, Tur-Kasper I, Amar A, Cohen I, Sharon R, Abecassis R, Levine C, Cohen T, Albert E. Histocompatibility determinants in Israeli Jewish patients with coeliac disease: population and family study. Tissue Antigens 1981;17:313-22.
13 Mearin ML, Bouquet I, Mourad N, Schoorel E, Sinaasappel M, Biemond I, Schreuder AThM, Peña AS, van Gelderen HH, van Rood JJ. HLA-DR antigens and phenotypes in Dutch coeliac children and their families. Clin Gen 1985;27:45-50.
14 Herrera M, Chertkoff L, Palavecino E, Mota A, Guala MC, Fainboim L, Satz ML. Restriction fragment length polymorphism in HLA class II gens of Latin-American Caucasian celiac disease patients. Hum Immunol 1989;26:272-80.
15 Tosi R, Tanigaki N, Polanco I, De Marchi M, Woodrow SC, Hetzel PhA. A radioimmunoassay typing study of non DQw2 associated coeliac disease. Clin Immunol Immunopathol 1986;39:168-72.
16 Hurley CK, Gregersen P, Steiner M, Bell J, Hartzman R, Nepom G, Silver J, Johnson AH. Polymorphism of the HLA-D region in American blacks. A DR3 haplotype generated by recombination. J Immunol 1988;140:885-92.
17 Bontrop RE, Baas EJ, Otting N, Schreuder GHT, Giphart MJ. Molecular diversity of HLA-DQ. DQ-alpha and -beta chain isoelectric point differences and their relation to serologically defined HLA-DQ allospecificities. Immunogenetics 1987;25:305-12.
18 Howell MD, Austin RK, Kelleher D, Nepom GT, Kagnoff M. An HLA-D region restriction fragment length polymorphism associated with celiac disease. J Exp Med 1986;164:333-8.
19 Karr RW, Gregersen PK, Obata F, Goldberg D, Maccari J, Alber C, Silver J. Analysis of DR β and DQ β chain cDNA clones from a DR7 haplotype. J Immunol 1986;137:2886-90.
20 Baur MP, Neugebauer M, Deppe H, Sigmund M, Luton T, Mayr WR, Albert ED. Population analysis on the basis of deduced haplotypes from random families. In: Histocompatibility testing 1984;pp 333-41. Eds. ED Albert, MP Baur, WR Mayr. Springer Verlag, Berlin.
21 Howell MD, Smith JR, Austin RK, Kelleher D, Nepom GT, Volk B, Kagnoff MF. An extended HLA-D region haplotype associated with celiac disease. Proc Natl Acad Sci 1988;85:222-6.
22 Bugawan T, Horn GT, Long CM, Mickelson E, Hansen JA, Ferrara GB, Angelini G, Erlich HA. Analysis of HLA-DP allelic sequences polymorphisms using the in vitro enzymatic NDA amplification of DP-α and DP-β loci. J Immunol 1988;141:4024-30.
23 Bugawan TL, Angelini G, Larrick J, Auriccio S, Ferrara GB, Erlick HA. A combination of a particular HLA-DP β allele and an HLA-DQ heterodimer confers susceptibility to coeliac disease. Nature 1989;339:470-3.
24 Brown JH, Jardetzky Th, Saper MA, Samraovi B, Bjorkman PJ, Wiley DC. A hypothetical model of the foreign antigen binding site of class II histocompatibility molecules. Nature 1988;332:845-50.
25 Rosenberg WMC, Wordsworth BP, Jewell DP, Bell JI. A locus telomeric to HLA-DPB encodes

susceptibility to coeliac disease. Immunogenetics 1989;30:307-10.
26 Scott H, Solheim BG, Brandtzaeg P, Thorsby E. HLA-DR like antigens in the epithelium of the human small intestine. Scand J Immunol 1981;12:77-82.
27 Arnaud Batandier F, Cerf-Bensussan N, Amsellem R, Schmitz J. Increased HLA-DR expression by enterocytes in children with celiac disease. Gastroenterology 1986;91:1205-12.
28 Ciclitira PJ, Nuluger SM, Ellis HJ, Evans DJ. The effect of gluten on HLA-DR in the small intestinal epithelium of patients with coeliac disease. Clin Exp Immunol 1986;63:101-4.
29 Marley NJE, MacArthey JC, Ciclitira PJ. HLA-DR, <-DP and <-DQ expression in the small intestine of patients with coeliac disease. Clin Exp Immunol 1987;70:386-93.
30 Sarles J, Gorvel JP, Olive D, Maroux S, Mawas C, Giraud I. Subcellular localization of class I (A,B,C) and class II (DR and DQ) MHC antigens in jejunal epithelium of children with coeliac disease. J Paed Gastroenterol Nutr 1987;6:51-6.
31 Tshibassu M, Geboes K, Eggermont E, Desmet V. Jejunal mucosa lymphoid cell subsets and the expression of major histocompatibility complex antigens in children. Eur J Pediatr 1987;146:251-6.
32 Kelly J, Weir DG, Faighery C. Differential expression of HLA-D gene products in the normal and coeliac small bowel. Tissue Antigens 1988;29:151-60.
33 Schweizer JJ, Mearin ML, Peña AS, Offerhaus GJA, Dreef EJ, Roep BO, Bontrop RE, Dooren LJ, Lamers CBHW, Hoedemaeker PhJ. HLA-DQ specific alleles strongly associated with coeliac disease are expressed at the small intestinal level in patients suffering from coeliac disease and in HLA-matched controls. In preparation.
34 Bonamico M, Mazzilli MC, Morellini M, Vania A, Carpino F, Nicotra MR, Natili PG. Expression of class II MHC antigens in the intestinal epithelium of pediatric celiac disease. J Paed Gastroenterol Nutr 1989;9:269-75.
35 Sette A, Buus S, Colon S, Smith JA, Miles C, Grey HM. Structural characteristics of an antigen required for its interaction with Ia and recognition by T cells. Nature 1987;328:395-9.
36 Teh HS, Kisielow P, Scott B, Kishi H, Vematsu Y, Blüthmann H, Boehmer H. Thymic major histocompatibility complex antigens and the α/β T-cell receptor determine the CD4/CD8 phenotype of T cells. Nature 1988;335:229-33.
37 Strober W. The influence of histocompatibility genes on the pathogenesis of gluten sensitive enteropathy. In: The genetics of coeliac disease 1981;pp:183-93. RB McConell Ed. Lancaster MTP Press.
38 Gallagher RB, Feighery C, Weir DG, Kelly CP, Whelan CA. Studies on the interaction between α-gliadin and HLA and T-cell receptor molecules in coeliac disease. Clin Exp Immunol 1988;74:413-18.
39 Bland P. MHC class II expression by the gut epithelium. Immunol Today 1988;9:174-8.

A CIS- OR TRANSASSOCIATED DQ HETERODIMER PREDISPOSES TO THE GLUTEN SENSITIVE ENTEROPATHY SEEN IN COELIAC DISEASE AND DERMATITIS HERPETIFORMIS.

M.A. Hall, J.S.S. Lanchbury, W.J. Bolsover, K.I. Welsh, P.J. Ciclitira.
Molecular Immunogenetics Laboratory, UMDS, Guy's Hospital, London and Division of Pharmacology, UMDS, St Thomas's Hospital, London, UK.

In order to address the question of a common genetic link predisposing to the enteropathy seen in both dermatitis herpetiformis (DH) and coeliac disease (CD), we have investigated HLA DR, DQ and DP associations by restriction fragment length genotyping in 80 CD patients, 23 DH patients with gluten sensitive enteropathy and 53 controls.
HLA-DQw2 is present in 95% CD patients (p=0.001), 100% DH patients (p=1.7 x 10-7) and in 40% controls. Significant secondary associations are seen with HLA-DR3 (90% in CD (p=0.001), 91% in DH (p=1.9 x 10-7) and 28% in controls) and DPw1 (40% in CD (p=0.001), 39% in DH (p=0.008) and 11% in controls).
DPw1 determined by RFLP was verified using DPB1 amplified DNA and oligonucleotide probes specific for the DPw1 associated DPB1 gene. The RFLP-assigned DPw1 genotype corresponded closely to the binding pattern of the sequence specific oligonucleotide probes. This DPw1 association is a result of linkage disequilibrium with B8 & DR3, and it is this haplotype that is highly represented in CD en DH, 42% of CD and 43% of DH DR3a haplotypes are extended to DPw1 versus 24% control DR3a haplotypes (p=0.003). 36% CD patients and 30% DH patients versus 4% controls are DR3,7 heterozygotes (p=0.001).
It is likely that HLA class II genes directly influence the immune response leading to mucosal damage in both CD and DH. The critical HLA molecule most likely to be involved is a specific DQα/DQβ heterodimer, encoded in cis arrangement in DR3 haplotypes or in trans in a DR3,7 or DR5,7 genotype. 93% of CD and 100% of DH patients (32% controls) are capable of expressing this molecule.

INTRODUCTION

The discovery that CD was associated with genes encoded within the HLA locus of the major histocompatibility complex (MHC) represented a major advance in the attempt to define the exact components of the genetic susceptibility to CD. HLA class II molecules bind specific antigen peptides and regulate immune responses. Identification of the precise HLA molecule, the antigenic component and the regulatory T-cell network represents a major challenge in understanding the pathogenesis of CD.
The common classical form of dermatitis herpetiformis (DH) is characterised by an itchy blistering skin eruption and granular IgA deposits at the dermoepidermal junction in an area not involved with the rash. Classical DH patients may exhibit gluten sensitive enteropathy, and the disease is associated with particular HLA-class I and class II antigens.
Although most patients with the classical form of DH have no overt gastrointestinal

M. L. Mearin and C. J. J. Mulder (eds.), Coeliac Disease, 35–41.

symptoms, gastrointestinal morphology is essentially identical to that seen in patients with ordinary CD, albeit less severe and more patchy (1). In order to address the question of a common genetic link predisposing to the enteropathy seen in both DH and CD, we have investigated HLA-DR, -DQ and -DP associations by restriction fragment length genotyping in 89 CD patients, 23 DH patients and 64 controls. Full length DRB, DQA, DQB, DPA and DPB cDNA probes were employed for the analyses. For DRB and DQB genotyping the restriction enzyme used was Taq I since it gave the most informative polymorphisms. The restriction enzyme Msp I was employed with Taq I for DP genotyping. The genotypes assigned by RFLP analysis were compared to the DRB alleles assigned using a group of sequence specific oligonucleotides (SSO's) directed at polymorphic regions of DRB locus genes amplified in a polymerase chain reaction (PCR) using DRB specific primers.

HLA DQw2 is present in 97.5% CD patients ($p<0.00001$), 100% DH patients ($p=1.7$ x 10-7) and in 45.3% controls. Significant secondary associations are seen with HLA-DR3 (87.5% in CD ($p<0.000001$), 91% in DH ($p=1.9$ x 10-7) and 21.9 % controls) and DPw1 (40% in CD ($p=0.001$), 39% in DH ($p=0.008$) and 11% in controls). A full representation of the results is shown in Tables I to III.

TABLE I RFLP DEFINED DR, DQ AND DP GENOTYPE FREQUENCIES IN COELIAC DISEASE PATIENTS AND CONTROLS

HLA-DR genotype	**CD (n=80)**	**controls (n=64)**
DR1	3.8 (3)	21.9 (14)
DR2	17.5 (14)	37.5 (24)
DR3a	87.5 (70)	21.9 (14)
DR4	10.0 (8)	28.1 (18)
DR5	7.5 (6)	12.5 (8)
DRw6	6.3 (5)	32.8 (21)
DR7b	45.0 (36)	26.6 (17)
HLA-DQ genotype		
DQw1	26.3 (21)	71.9 (46)
DQw2c	97.5 (78)	45.3 (29)
DQw3	20.0 (16)	45.3 (29)
HLA-DP genotype		**controls (n=53)**
DPw1d	40.0 (32)	11.0 (6)
DPw2	12.5 (10)	25.0 (13)
DPw3/6	50.0 (40)	49.0 (26)
DPw4	60.0 (48)	81.0 (43)
DPw5	9.0 (7)	9.0 (5)
DPCp63	11.0 (9)	6.0 (3)

a: Fisher's p=4 x 10-16; b: Fisher's p=0.02; c: Fisher's p=1.4 X 10-13; d: Fisher's p=0.0002.

TABLE II HLA CLASS II GENOTYPE AND OLIGONUCLEOTIDE DATA IN DERMATITIS HERPETIFORMIS

	HLA class II genotype			Oligonucleotide data			
Name	DR	DQ	DP	258C	401D	402D	849D
FB	3,7	2a2b	1,1	+	+	+	-
JB	3,7	2a2b	1,4	+	+	+	-
DC1	2,3	1b2a	1,4	+	+	+	-
JC1	3,3	2a2a	1,4	+	+	+	-
JC2	3,7	2a2b	4,3/6	-	+	-	-
DC2	2,3	1b2a	4,3/6	-	-	-	-
DC3	2,3	1a2a	1,2	+	+	+	-
MC	5,7	2b3b	4,4	-	-	-	-
EF	2,3	1b2a	1,4	+	+	+	-
EG	3,w8	2a3a	4,4	-	-	-	-
KH	3,w6	1a2a	2,5	-	-	-	-
DH	3,w6	1b2a	4,4	-	-	-	-
MJ	3,7	2a2b	1,5	+	+	+	-
PK	3,7	2a2b	3/6,Cp63	-	+	-	-
MK	3,w6	1a2a	4,3/6	-	+	-	-
SM	3,w6	1b2a	4,3/6,5	-	+	-	-
AR	3,7	2a2b	2,4	-	-	-	-
BR	2,3	1b2a	4,3/6,5	-	+	-	-
RS	5,7	2b3b	4,4	-	-	-	-
CS	2,3	1b2a	4,4	-	-	-	-
JS	3,4	2a3a	1,2	+	+	+	-
BT	3,3	2a2a	4,3/6,5	-	-	-	-
WT	1,3	1a2a	1,4	+	+	+	-

DRB allele assignment using DRB SSO's has shown that in 75 CD patients and 23 DH patients the allele assignment corresponded exactly to the RFLP defined genotypes with only four exceptions (data not shown). Since the reactivity patterns of the SSO's for defined alleles is the same in the disease patients and controls, it is unlikely that there is a disease specific allele. The four discrepancies may be ascribed to novel allele sequences, although this has not yet been confirmed.

The application of PCR and SSO hybridisation has had a great impact on the characterisation of DPB alleles as well as DRB alleles. Six cellularly-defined allotypes designated DPw1-6 have been well described, and a number of local definitions such as Cp63 and CDP-HEI also exist (2-4). RFLP analysis has shown that certain restriction fragments correlate significantly with one or more cellularly-defined DPw specificities (5,6). Bugawan have shown that specific DPB1 sequences correlate with the classical PLT-defined DPw types. Sequence analysis of the DPB locus has resulted in the definition of 21 DPB1 sequence variants (7,8) showing that the polymorphism of DPB1 is more extensive than was previously recognised. Molecular definition of DP polymorphism has enabled a number of previously blank cellular specificities to be associated with novel DPB1 sequences.

TABLE III COMPARISON OF HLA DR, DQ AND DP PHENOTYPE FREQUENCIES AMONG DERMATITIS HERPETIFORMIS PATIENTS AND CONTROLS.

Fosher's p values, relative risks (RR) and etiological fractions (ef) are given below for statistically significant positive associations.

DR Type	% DH (n=23)	% Controls (n=53)
1	-	26 (14)
2	26 (6)	30 (16)
3a	91 (21)	28 (15)
4	4 (1)	28 (15)
5	9 (2)	13 (7)
w6	17 (4)	24 (13)
7	35 (8)	28 (15)
w8	4 (1)	6 (3)
DQ Type		
w1	48 (11)	66 (35)
w2b	100 (23)	40 (21)
w3	17 (4)	47 (25)
DP Type		
w1c	39 (9)	11 (6)
w2	17 (4)	25 (13)
w3/6	26 (6)	49 (26)
w4	70 (16)	81 (43)
w5	9 (2)	9 (5)
Cp63	4 (1)	6 (3)

a: p=1.9 x 10-7 , RR=22, EF=0.88; b: p=1.7 x 10-7 , RR=68, EF=1.00; c: p=0.008, RR= 4.8, EF=0.32.

This approach to DNA typing of DP antigens allows a more accurate analysis of the significance of DP polymorphism in disease studies. To confirm the accuracy of the RFLP defined DPw1 genotype, oligonucleotide probes targeting specific DPw1-associated DPB1 sequences were hybridised to amplified DNA from the second exon of the DPB1 gene (Table IV). The DPw1 genotype assigned by RFLP analysis corresponds exactly to the pattern of hybridisation of the oligonucleotides assigned to the DPB1 allele in all the DPw1 positive DH patients and in 29/32 of the DPw1 CD patients. Three CD patients positive for the DPw1 RFLPs lacked the DPw1 beta chain sequence. The association however between DPw1 and CD remained. The distribution of oligonucleotide defined DPw1 in CD and DH revealed that DPw1 was only present in those individuals who type HLA-DR3a positive. The DR3a subtype is usually associated with B8,DR3 (data not shown). Two alternative explanations for the coincidence of DR3a and DPw1 in CD and DH patients can be made. First, DPw1 may be raised in CD as a marker conferring increased susceptibility specifically within a DR3a phenotypic background, or secondly there may be a DR3a-DPw1 extended haplotype which strongly predisposes to CD. Data from DR3a selected controls shows that 24% are DPw1 compared with 5% non-DR3a controls typing as DPw1 (Fisher's p=0.03). These data suggest that there is a significant asociation between DR3a and DPw1 in the control population, indicating that a proportion of normal extended DR3a haplotypes include DPw1. This extended haplotype also appears particularly prevalent among DR3a positive CD and DH patients. Compared with 7/29 (24%) controls selected for DR3a positivity 29/69 (42%) DR3a CD patients and 9/21 (43%) DR3a DH patients typed as DPw1. This difference is not significant (Fisher's p=0.07), suggesting that although the haplotype is more highly represented in the disease groups, the increase is not significant compared to controls (10).

TABLE IV DPB1 AMPLIFICATION PRIMERS AND SEQUENCE SPECIFIC OLIGONUCLEOTIDE PROBES DEFINING DPW1 ASSOCIA TED NUCLEOTIDE SEQUENCES

Name	Sequence	Amino Acids	DPB allele Specificity
259C	5'CCCCTCCCCGCAGAGAATTAC		5' Primer
257C	5'AAGCCCTCACTCACCTCGGCG		3' Primer
258C	5'TACGTGTACCAGGGACGGC	7-12	1,15,18
401D	5'GTCTGCATACCCTGTCC	74-78	1,3,7,8,9,10,12,14
402D	5'AGGAGTACGCGCGCTTC	34-38	1,11,13,15
849D	5'GAGCTGGTCGGGCCCAT	84-88	15,18

In our population it has been shown that it is a DR3a haplotype that includes DPw1 which is significantly raised in both CD and DH. PCR amplification of the DPB1 second exon and hybridisation with SSO's has shown DPB alleles 1,3 and 4.2 to be raised in different ethnic groups with CD (7). It is likely that all three alleles are in linkage disequilibrium with DR3 (9), indicating that different DR3 extended haplotypes are represented in different CD and DH populations. There is firm evidence for a shared genetic basis for the gluten sensitive enteropathy seen in CD and DH. The strongest clue so far to understanding the shared pathogenesis is the mapping of susceptibility to the HLA class II region of the MHC. This region contains genes coding for heterodimeric transmembrane glycoproteins which determine the magnitude and specificity of immune responses (11). CD and DH share a similar immunopathology, namely T lymphocyte infiltration into the small intestinal intraepithelial layer and increased levels of anti-gliadin antibodies. It is reasonable, therefore, to suppose that HLA class II genes directly influence specific immune responses leading to the characteristic mucosal damage. The first task is to identify the HLA class II locus responsible. This is complicated by the extreme linkage disequilibrium shown by the A1 B8 DR3 DQw2 haplotype asociated with both CD and DH. Although CD and DH are significantly associated with DR3, DQw2 and DPw1, the strongest association is with DQw2 which must be considered the candidate allele for DH (12). The increase in DR3 and DPw1 can be explained by their existence on an extended haplotype which is highly represented in the disease population. This conclusion is strengthened by recent reports that the HLA-molecule most consistently associated with CD is a specific DQw2 DQ alpha/beta heterodimer encoded in cis arrangement on a DR3 haplotype (13,14). Since the same DQ alpha allele is also shared between DR3 and DR5 haplotypes, an identical transassociated DQ alpha/DQ beta dimer could be expressed by DR5,7 individuals. Our data on DH fits this model perfectly. The two patients who do not type as DR3 are DR5,7 and are capable of expressing the transassociated DQ alpha/DQ beta dimer. Thus 100% of DH patients (p=5.8 x 10-11) and 91% CD patients (p=4 x 10-17) in contrast to 25% controls have the potential to express the dimer in cis or trans configuration, and is therefore a stronger marker for disease susceptibility than DQw2. Since the pathogenesis of both CD and DH involve gluten intolerance, one could speculate that the shared association with a DQ alpha/DQ beta dimer predisposes to the enteropathy in both diseases, and that the severity of the mucosal damage and the skin lesions associated with DH are the results of other interacting genetic loci and/or environmental factors.

This work was funded by the Wellcome Trust, The Coeliac Trust and St.Thomas Hospital Research (endowments) Committee.

REFERENCES

1 Scott BB, Losowsky MS. Patchiness and mucosal abnormality in coeliac disease (CD) and dermatitis herpetiformis. Gut 1975;16:393.
2 Shaw S, Pollack MS, Payne SM, Johnson AH. HLA-linked B cell antigens of a new segregant series: Population and family studies of the SB antigens. Hum Immunol 1985;1:145.
3 Nose Y, Nakatsuji T, Tsuji K, Reinsmoen NL. A new DP (SB) specificity (Cp63) defined in Japanese and caucasian cell populations by cloned PLT cells. Hum Immunol 1985;13:145.
4 Odum N, Hartzman RJ, Jakobsen BK, Morling N, Platz P, Jakobsen B, Svejgaard A. The HLA DP polymorphism in Denmark investigated by local and international PLT reagents. Definitions of two "new" DP antigens. Tissue Antigens 1986;28:105.
5 Hyldig-Nielsen JJ, Morling N, Odum N, Ryder LP, Platz P, Jakobsen B, Svejgaard A. Restriction fragment length polymorphism of the HLA-DP subregion and correlations to HLA-DP phenotypes. Proc Natl Acad Sci USA 1987;84:1644.
6 Maeda M, Inoko H, Ando A, Uryu N, Nagata Y, Tsuji K. HLA-DP typing by analysis of DNA restriction fragment length polymorphism in the HLA-DPB subregion. Hum Immunol 1988;21:239.
7 Bugawan TL, Angelini G, Larrick J, Auricchio S, Ferrara GB, Erlich HA. A combination of a particular HLA-DPB allele and an HLA-DQ heterodimer confers susceptibility to coeliac disease. Nature 1989;339:470.
8 Bugawan TL, Horn GT, Long CM, Mickelson E, Hansen JA, Ferrara GB, Angelini G, Erlich HA. Analysis of HLA-DP allelic sequence polymorphism using the in vitro enzymatic DNA amplification of DP-A and DP-B loci. J Immunol 1988;141:4024.
9 Rosenberg WMC, Wordsworth BP, Jewell DP, Bell JI. A locus telomeric to HLA-DPB encodes susceptibility to coeliac disease. Immunogenetics 1989;30:307.
10 Hall MA, Lanchbury JSS, Bolsover WJ, Welsk KI, Ciclitira PJ. Celiac disease is associated with an extended HLA-DR3 haplotype which includes DPw1. Hum Immunol 1990;27:220.

11 Kaufman JF, Auffray C, Korman AJ, Shackelford DA, Strominger J. The class II molecules of the human and murine major histocompatibility complex. Cell 1984;36:1.
12 Hall MA, Lanchbury JSS, Bolsover WJ, Welsh KI, Ciclitira PJ. The HLA association with dermatitis herpetiformis is accounted for by a cis- or transassociated DQ heterodimer. Gut in press.
13 Roep BO, Bontrop RE, Pena AS, van Eggermond MCJA, van Rood JJ, Giphart MJ. An HLA-DQ alpha allele identified at DNA and protein level is strongly associated with coeliac disease. Hum Immunol 1988;23:271.
14 Sollid LM, Markussen G, Ek J, Gjerde H, Vartdal F, Thorsby E. Evidence for a primary association of celiac disease to a particular HLA DQ alpha/beta heterodimer. J Exp Med 1989;169:345.

NONHUMAN PRIMATES AS ANIMAL MODELS FOR COELIAC DISEASE: APPROACH AND FEASIBILITY.

R.E. Bontrop, Institute of Applied Radiobiology and Immunology TNO, Primate Center, Lange Kleiweg 151, 2280 HV, Rijswijk, The Netherlands.

Within the human caucasoid population Coeliac Disease (CD) shows an extremely strong association (RR = 158) with a particular MHC class II DQαβ dimer. However, it is not yet clear whether this dimer itself plays a major role in the onset or prolongation of CD. Alternatively, it can formally not be excluded that the DQαβ dimer may be a marker within the caucasoid population found in close genetic linkage with yet unkwown CD associated gene(s). Linkage disequilibria are known to differ within distinct human ethnic populations due to recombinations. For that reason, if one wants to pinpoint an immune response gene one should study patients from a different ethnic background. However, it should be well established that the causal antigen and disease studied are identical within these different populations. Such a strategy even could be extrapolated to the level of nonhuman primate species since it is known that these species may suffer from the same type of diseases as man. Although there exists a close phytogenetic relationship between man, great apes and monkey species the disease associated MHC immune response genes may exhibit sequence variation due to separate evolution. On first sight this can be considered as a disadvantage. In our opinion, such types of MHC-transspecies disease associated immune response genes exhibiting a minor degree of heterogeneity may be extremely helpful in determining the relevant disease associated epitope.

INTRODUCTION

From a phylogenetic and evolutionary point of view, the great ape and monkey species are more closely related to man than any other experimental animal. This close relationship is reflected by the observation that a large amount of monoclonal antibodies originally raised against polymorphic and frame-work human MHC and Cluster of Differentiation markers do crossreact with nonhuman primate cells. For this reason, nonhuman primates may provide excellent experimental animal models to study autoimmunity and infectious diseases. Apart from this, it has been documented that distinct species may exhibit differential tissue distributions for the same type of antigens. For instance, activated mouse T cells do not express MHC class II molecules whereas human and nonhuman primate T cells certainly express those type of heterodimers. This example, again emphasizes why one may choose for nonhuman primate species as an experimental animal model instead for rodent species. Experimental animal models may especially be usefull in those situations in which one wants to study the mechanism of a disease. Detailed knowledge gained on the biological role of MHC immune response genes and interaction with the T cell receptor (TCR) complex may provide insight how one has to manipulate the immune system to prevent the onset of certain types of immunological disorders. Of course, it is of crucial importance to know exactly the agent or pathogen that causes the disease. CD would be an ideal candidate for such studies since in the case of this

M. L. Mearin and C. J. J. Mulder (eds.), Coeliac Disease, 43–49.

disease the antigen is known and the input of genetic factors has been documented in man.

HUMAN IMMUNOGENETICS OF COELIAC DISEASE

CD is characterized by small intestinal mucosal athrophy elicited by ingestion of wheat gluten in genetically susceptible individuals (1). However, less than 0.2% of the individuals which have the disease associated MHC genes develop CD despite the dietary intake of wheat (2). Interestingly, disease is not always concordant among monozygotic twins (3,4). Based on those observations it has been postulated that additional environmental factors may play a role in the pathogenesis of CD. The possible influence of human adenovirus in the onset of CD has been reported (5). The task of the immune system is to mount an immune response against foreign pathogens like viruses and bacteria.

One of the mechanisms involved in the elimination of pathogens is the production of antibodies. HLA class II molecules are thought to function in the regulation of such an immune response by presenting foreign antigen segments to regulator T cells resulting in antigen-dependent B cell activation. Unlike B cells, which may bind soluble antigen directly by their immunoglobulins, T cells recognize antigen or processed antigen only in the context of a self MHC structure, a phenomenon known as MHC restriction.

Nowadays, it is generally accepted that peptides or degraded antigen particles can directly bind to MHC class II structures (6-8). The hallmark of the HLA-system is its extensive allelic polymorphism thought to reflect the need to respond to a vartiety of antigens as wide as possible, thereby minimizing the chance of non-responsiveness due to a hole of the repertoire. In principle, one can find a hole in the repertoire both for MHC molecules and T cell receptors. However, a striking difference between these two genetic systems is that the TCR complex displays its polymorphism within the individual whereas the MHC exhibits its abundant allelic polymorphism for the major part within the population. For that reason, a hole in the repertoire for the T cell receptor (TCR) complex is not easily found (9).

Holes in the MHC repertoire are rather frequent observed in the case of small peptides. Failures to present antigen are more difficult detected in the case of complex polypeptides. On the other hand, it is not unlikely that at the present time one cannot detect MHC molecules which fail to present antigens derived from micro-organisms which once (or still) represented a serious threat to mankind. In other words, individuals originally present within the population which could not respond properly to some pathogenic threats may have been selected out long ago.

One of the intriguing phenomena in HLA biology is the observation that certain HLA-class II alleles seem to be associated with an increased risk to develop certain diseases. The strength of the association or the extent to which an individual carrying a particular class II allele is more likely to contract a disease is called relative risk (RR) which indicates how many more times the disease occurs among individuals having the allele as compared to those lacking the allele. It has been reported that the susceptibility genes for CD may be associated with HLA-B8, -DR3, -DR5, -DR7, -DQw2 and some HLA-DP specificities (10-16).

The presence of the HLA-B8, -DR3, -DQw2 and -DPw1 specificities is for the major part explained by the overrepresentation of the HLA-A1-B8-DR3-DQw2-DPw1 extended haplotype in CD patients (16).

CIS AND TRANS GENE COMPLEMENTATION.

Evidence for gene complementation of class II molecules was originally found in the murine system by the demonstration that hybrid class II molecules could exist in F1-animals (17, 18). In man, transgene complementation has been shown in the case of HLA-DQ heterozygotes (19, 20), meaning that the polymorphic class II DQ alpha chain in principle can associate with the DQ beta chains encoded by the paternal and maternal haplotypes.
The strongest RR value to develop CD seems to be associated with a particular class II DQ alpha-beta chain dimer (12, 14). This class II dimer may be encoded in cis by the HLA-A1-B8-DQw2-DPw1 haplotype or in a trans fashion when the DQ alpha chain is encoded by HLA-DR3-DQw2 or HLA-DR5-DQw3 positive cells whereas the relevant DQ beta chain is derived from the complementary haplotype carrying the HLA-DR7-DQw2 specificity. This trans complementation most likely explains the relative high percentage of HLA-DR3 negative but HLA-DR5,7 positive coeliac patients. These data suggest that a specific DQ heterodimer may be involved in the genetic risk to develop CD.

QUANTITATIVE ASPECTS OF MHC-CLASS II EXPRESSION.

Quantitative variation in class II antigen expression was again first noticed in the mouse. It was shown that such variation could lead to profound alterations in immune responsiveness (21, 22). Quantitative variation in the expression of class II molecules was reported to account for, or at least influence, "cis-trans" or gene dosage effects in responsiveness to antigen (23). This phenomenon also may explain some examples of non-responsiveness in the non-responder strains of mice found in Ir-gene studies (24). Especially dendritic cells seem to be characterized by a high density of surface Ia molecules (25).
In this context it has been reported that a murine specific immune response defect could be abolished by immunization with dendritic cells (26) indicating that there exists a close relationship between antigen presenting capacity and density of surface class II molecules (27). In the case of the human MHC, quantitative variation in HLA class II expression results in functional consequences too (28).

THE TRANS-SPECIES HYPOTHESIS FOR THE GENERATION OF MHC POLYMORPHISM.

There is accumulating evidence that some MHC alleles predate speciation (29-33). In other words, man, great apes and different monkey species have inhereted the same alleles from a common ancestor. These ancestral MHC alleles have undergone separate developments after speciation, most times induced by means of point mutations resulting in the fact that distinct species like man, chimpanzee, gorilla, orangutan, rhesus monkey etc. express related alleles that display a low degree of aminoacid variations. This convergent evolution of MHC polymorphism explains why some MHC alleles of different species are more related to each other than the MHC alleles from one species itself. However it should be taken into account that when the evolutionary gap becomes larger that the degree of sequence similarity diminishes.

The implication of these findings is that from a MHC point of view, nonhuman primates are the ideal species to study T cell mediated autoimmune diseases. The trans-species MHC sequence variation occuring among ancestral alleles can be used as a big advantage. If one is studying the same type of disease, caused by the same type of pathogen, combined relative risk and sequence comparison studies may enable to pinpoint the disease related epitope.

However, not all MHC-class II sequence variation necessarilly has functional implications. It has been documented that trans species MHC polymorphisms can be translated into functional data, despite the fact that the MHC class II alleles involved display a relative high degree of sequence heterogeneity (34).

LINKAGE DISEQUILIBRIUM.

As stated above separate MHC alleles originating from one ancestral allele may have been altered in evolution by point mutations. Other genetic mechanisms that have been claimed to be involved in the generation of MHC class II polymorphism are gene conversion or intragenic crossing-over.

The mechanism generating probably the majority of the MHC associated polymorphisms is homologous crossing-over influencing the combination of different alleles on one chromosome. The tendency for alleles at different loci to occur on the same haplotype more often than expected by chance is called linkage disequilibrium.

It has been proposed that selective advantage may explain why certain linkage disequilibria are frequently observed within the human population. Some of these may reflect the presence of ancestral haplotypes (35). Linkage disequilibria appear to differ among ethnic populations and may have been influenced by climate (36) or pathogenic factors (37). Natural selection may give rise to situations at which only a small spectrum of the original total of HLA-antigens has remained at a certain topographic area. Therefore linkage disequilibrium or gene arrangement of polymorphic genes is not a status quo situation but reflects a fixed moment in evolution. As a consequence some MHC associated diseases may be completely absent or rare in different populations of a species. In conclusion linkage disequilibria are differing among distinct human ethnic populations and it is likely that gene arrangement of MHC alleles also exhibit variety in distinct species. As a consequence studies on the detection of immune response genes within different ethnic populations and species may exclude the possibility that data are difficult to interprete due to the over-representation of extended haplotypes.

COELIAC DISEASE MODELS IN NON-HUMAN PRIMATES: APPROACH AND FEASABILITY.

Chronic diarrhea and weight loss are common clinical signs often observed in

non-human primate colonies. The cause for these observations remains usually unidentified. Recently, it has been documented that gluten-sensitive enteropathy may occur in cynomolgus monkeys (38). The malabsorption syndrome and the villous atrophy disappeared when grain products were removed from the diet.
It is of major interest to determine the MHC class II DQ alleles of this particular animal. Sequence studies on the MHC DQA1 alleles of cynomolgous monkeys demonstrated that the equivalent of the HLA-DQA1 allele which is strongly associated with coeliac disease is present within cynomolgous monkeys too (manuscript in preparation). Another significant observation is that in the ITRI-TNO, primate center rhesus monkey colony, which counts roughly a 1000 individuals, the equivalent of the CD associated DQA1 allele appears to virtually absent or at least extremely rare. A study performed on another population of rhesus monkeys demonstrated the presence of this particular MHC-DQA1 allele within the rhesus monkey population. At present we are investigating whether the origin or other facts such as diet may have influenced the MHC class II repertoire in our rhesus monkey colony.

REFERENCES.

1 Van de Kamer JH, Weijers HA, Dicke WK. An investigation into the injurious constituents of wheat in connection with their action on patients with coeliac disease. Acta Paediatr. 1958; 42:2232.
2 Albert ED, Harms K, Wank R, Steinbauer-Rosenthal and Scholz S. Segregation analysis of HLA-antigens and haplotypes in 50 families of patients with coeliac disease. Transplant Proc. 1973; 5:1785.
3 Hoffman HN, Wollaeger EE, Greenberg E. Discordance for nontropical sprue (adult coeliac disease) in a monozygotic twin pair. Gastroenterology. 1966; 51:36.
4 Walker-Smith JA. Discordance for childhood coeliac disease in monozygotic twins. Gut 1973; 14:374.
5 Kagnoff MF, Austin RK, Hubert JJ, Bernadin JE, Kasarda DD. Possible role for a human adenovirus in the pathogenesis of coeliac disease. J Exp Med. 1984; 160:1544.
6 Babbitt BP, Allen PM, Matsueda G, Haber E, Unanue ER. Antigenic competitions at the level of antigen - Ia complexes involved in T-cell recognition. Nature. 1985; 317:359.
7 Buus S, Sette A, Colon SM, Miles C, Grey HM. The relation between major histocompatibility (MHC) restriction and the capacity of Ia to bind immunogenic peptides. Science 1987; 235:1353.
8 Guillet JG, Lai M, Briner TJ, Smith JA, Gefter ML. Interaction of peptide antigens and class II major histocompatibility complex antigens. Nature 1986; 324:260.
9 Ogasawara K, Maloy WL, Schwartz RH. Failure to find a hole in the T cell repertoire. Nature. 1987; 325:450.
10 Keuning JJ, Peña AS, Van Leeuwen A, Van Hoff JP, Van Rood JJ. HLA-DW3 associated with Coeliac Disease. Lancet. 1976; i:506.
11 Tosi R, Vismara D, Tanigaki N, Ferrara GB, Cicimarra F, Buffolano W, Follo D, Auricchio S. Evidence that celiac disease is primarily associated with a DC allelic specificity. Clin Immunol Immunopathol. 1983; 28:395.
12 Sollid LM, Markussen G, Ek J, Gjerde H, Vartdal F, Thorsby E. Evidence for a primary association of Celiac Disease to a particular HLA-DQ α/β heterodimer. J Exp Med. 1989; 169:345.
13 Mearin ML, Biemond I, Peña AS, Polanco I, Vazquez C, Schreuder GMTh, De Vries RRP, van Rood JJ. HLA-DR phenotypes in Spanish coeliac children: their contribution to the understanding of the genetics of the disease. Gut. 1983; 24:532.
14 Roep BO, Bontrop RE, Peña AS, Van Eggermond MCJA, van Rood, JJ, Giphart MJ. An

HLA-DQ α allele identified at DNA and protein level is strongly associated with celiac disease. Hum Immunol. 1988; 23:271.
15 Niven MJ, Caffrey C, Sachs JA, Gasell PG, Gallegher RB, Kumar P, Hitman GA. Susceptibility to coeliac disease involves genes in HLA-DP region. Lancet 1987; ii:805.
16 Hall MA, Lanchbury JS, Bolsover WJ, Welsh KI, Ciclitira PJ. Celiac disease is associated with an extended HLA-DR3 haplotype which includes HLA-DPw1. Hum Immunol. 1990; 27:220.
17 Cook R, Vitetta E, Uhr J, Capra J. Structural studies on the murine Ia alloantigens. III tryptic peptide comparisons of allelic products of the l-E/c subregion. J Immunol. 1980; 124:1594.
18 Silver J, Swain SL, Hubert JJ. The small subunit of I-A subregion antigens determines the allospecificity recognized by a monoclonal antibody. Nature. 1980; 286:272.
19 Charron DJ, Lotteau V, Turmel P. Hybrid HLA-DQ antigens provide molecular evidence for gene trans-complementation. Nature. 1984; 312:157.
20 Giles RC, DeMars R, Chang CC, Capra JD. Allelic polymorphism and transassociations of molecules encoded by the HLA-DQ subregion. Proc Natl Acad Sci USA. 1985; 82:1776.
21 McNicholas JM, Murphy DB, Matis LA, Schwartz RH, Lerner EA, Janeway CA, Jones PP. Immune response gene function correlates with the expression of an Ia antigen. J Exp Med. 1982; 155:490.
22 Matis LA, Jones PP, Murphy DB, Hedrick SM, Lerner EA, Janeway CA, McNicolas JM, Schwartz RH. A quantitative defect in Ae:Eα complex expression causes a corresponding defect in antigen-presenting cell function. J Exp Med. 1982; 155:508.
23 Conrad PJ, Lerner EA, Murphy DB, Jones PP, Janeway CA. Differential expression of Ia glycoproteïn complexes in F1 hybrid mice detected with alloreactive cloned T cell lines. J Immunol. 1982; 129:2616.
24 Janeway CA, Bottomly K, Babich J, Conrad P, Conzen S, Jones B, Kaye J, Katz M, McVay L, Murphy DB, Tite J. Quantitative variation in Ia antigen expression plays a cental role in immune regulation. Immunol Today. 1984; 5:99.
25 Steinman RM, Gutchinov B, Witmer MD, Nussenzweig MC. Dendritic cells are the principal stimulators of the primary mixed leukocyte reactions in mice. J Exp Med. 1983; 157:613.
26 Boog CJP, Kast WM, Timmers HThM, Boes J, De Waal DP, Melief CJM. Abolition of specific immune response defect by immunization with dendritic cells. Nature. 1985; 318:59.
27 Matis LA, Glimcher LH, Paul WE, Schwartz RH. Magnitude of response of histocompatibility restricted T cell clones is a function of the products of the concentrations of antigen and Ia molecules. Proc Natl Acad Sci USA. 1983; 80:6019.
28 Bontrop R, Ottenhoff T, van Miltenburg R, Elferink D, De Vries R, Giphart M. Quantitative and qualitative differences in HLA-DR correlated with antigen presentation capacity. Eur J Immunol. 1986; 16:133.
29 Lawlor DA, Ward FE, Ennis PE, Jackson AP, Parham P. HLA-A and B polymorphisms predate the divergence of humans and chimpanzees. Nature. 1988; 335:268.
30 Mayer WE, Jonker M, Klein D, Ivanyi P, van Seventer G, Klein J. Nucleotide sequences of chimpanzee MHC class I alleles; evidence for transspecies mode of evolution. EMBO J. 1988; 7:2765.
31 Klein J. Origin of the major histocompatibility complex polymorphism: the trans species hypothesis. Hum Immunol. 1987; 19:155.
32 Bontrop RE, Otting N, Broos LAM, Noort MC, Kenter M, Jonker M. RFCP analysis of the HLA-, ChLA, and RhlA-DQ α chain region: conservation of restricions determinants in evolution. Immunogenetics. 1989; 30:432.
33 Fan W, Kasahara M, Gutknecht J, Klein D, Mayer WE, Jonker M, Klein J. Shared class Ii MHC polymorphisms between humans and chimpanzees. Hum Immunol. 1989; 26:107.
34 Bontrop RE, Elferink DG, Otting N, Jonker M, De Vries RRP. Major histocompatibility complex class II restricted antigen presentation across a species barrier: conservation of restriction determinants in evolution. J Exp Med. 1990;172:53.
35 Tokunaga K, Saueracker G, Kay PH, Christiansen FT, Anand R, Dawkins RL. Extensive deletions and insertions in different MHC supratypes detected by pulsed field gel electrophoresis. J Exp Med 1988; 168:933.

36 Piazza A, Menozzi P, Cavalli-Sforza LL.The HLA-A, B gene frequencies in the world: migration or selection. Hum Immunol 1980; 1:297.
37 De Vries RRP, Meera Khan P, Bernini LF, Van Lochem E, van Rood JJ. Genetic control of survival in epidemics. J Immunogenetics 1988; 18:503.
38 Wagner JD, Jerome CP, Adams MR. Gluten-sensitive enteropathy in a cynomolgus monkey. Lab Animal Science. 1988; 38:592.

T-CELL SUBPOPULATIONS IN INTESTINAL MUCOSA.

Thomas T MacDonald, Dept. of Paediatric Gastroenterology, St Bartholomews Hospital, London EC1A 7BE, UK.
Jo Spencer, Dept. of Histopathology, University College and Middlesex School of Medicine, London WC1E 6JJ, UK.

There is considerable T cell heterogeneity in normal and diseased human small bowel. Most studies have focussed on intraepithelial lymphocyte (IEL) subpopulations; changes in lamina propria T cells are less well documented. In normal intestine, of the CD3+ IEL, 80% are CD8+, 10% CD4+ and about 6% are CD4-, 8-. In addition there is a relatively large population of CD3-, 7+ IEL (5-25% of total IEL). About 50% of normal IEL are CD45RO+, and only a few are γδ TcR+. In untreated coeliac disease, there is a large increase in the percentage of CD3+,4-,8- IEL (10-65%), the CD3-, 7+ IEL disappear, and these is a dramatic increase in γδ TcR+ (30%) and CD45RO expression. The increase in γδ TcR+IEL appears to be specific for coeliac disease and persists even on a gluten-free diet. γδ TcR+ IEL use different V region genes from most blood γδ TcR+ T cells. While the significance of these changes in the pathogenesis of coeliac disease will only be elucidated when the function of IEL subpopulations is determined, the increase in γδ TcR+ IEL may be of some diagnostic importance.

INTRODUCTION

Although it has been realised for many years that the intestinal mucosa contains large numbers of lymphocytes, it is only in the last 10 years that these cells have been characterised in detail in normal and diseased mucosae. This has been achieved by the development and widespread use of immunohistochemistry using monoclonal antibodies to T cell surface markers. Compared to the large number of immunohistochemical studies, few functional studies on human gut lymphocytes have been reported. Since there is some doubt as to the origin of cells isolated from large pieces of human gut (Peyer's patch or lamina propria) and since these studies have failed to shed light on the pathogenesis of intestinal inflammation they will not be considered further. Here we would like to consider mucosal T cell subpopulations in normal intestine, intestine from patients with a flat mucosa (coeliac disease (CD) and tropical sprue) and the human fetus which gives the baseline populations in the absence of antigenic stimulation from the lumen. Discussion will be confined to the T cell populations of the lamina propria and epithelium.

T CELLS IN NORMAL LAMINA PROPRIA.

The benchmark paper of Janossy (1) established that within normal human gut there are marked differences in the T cell populations of the epithelium and lamina propria. Most of the T cells within the lamina propria are CD4+ with only a minority CD8+. Lamina propria macrophages are CD4+ and thus estimates of CD4+ cells in lamina propria will lead to an overestimate of the proportion of CD4+ T

M. L. Mearin and C. J. J. Mulder (eds.), Coeliac Disease, 51–56.

cells. Double staining of CD3+ cells with CD4 or CD8 has however confirmed that most lamina propria T cells are CD4+ (2). About half of the lamina propria T cells are CD45RA and half are CD45RO, indicating a mixed population of primary and secondary T cells (3). Lamina propria T cells differ from peripheral T cells in that most of them are Leu8-, a feature associated with helper rather than suppressor/ inducer function (4). Over 90% of lamina propria T cells use the αß T cell receptor (TcR), with γδ TcR+ cells only rarely seen in normal colonic or small bowel lamina propria (5). In the fetus, the T cells which populate the lamina propria from 14 weeks gestation are CD4+ (6).

T CELLS IN NORMAL EPITHELIUM.

Most of the T cells in small and large bowel epithelium are CD8+ (1). Less than 20% are CD4+. IEL are unusual in that most are CD5- (7,8). The monoclonal antibody HML-1 (9) stains 90% of IEL. It is believed that HML-1 recognises some form of activation marker on T cells, and consistent with this about half of IEL also stain with the late activation marker VLA-1 (10), and the same proportion are CD45R0+ (11). Recently it has been demonstrated that not all IEL are T cells. In normal individuals between 5 and 25% of IEL are CD3-,CD7+ (8,12). These cells are concentrated at the villus tips, but their function is unknown. Since these cells do not have a TcR they cannot respond to antigen.

Of the CD3+ IEL, most bear subset markers. But in normal bowel between 2 and 10% of the CD3+ IEL are CD4-,CD8- (12). T cells using the γδ TcR are not frequent in normal human gut epithelium (12,13), however 90% of them are CD8- (8,14). The effect of antigen on normal IEL populations can be studied using fetal material. IEL numbers in the fetus are about 25% of that in the adult (6). As in post-natal bowel, there are more CD8+ IEL than CD4+ IEL (6), however about 50% of fetal IEL are CD4-,CD8- (12). There are few CD3-, CD7+ fetal IEL. As would be expected with a large proportion of CD4-, 8- IEL, about 30% of fetal IEL are γδ TcR+ (5). Details of T cell subsets in lamina propria and epithelium are shown in Table I.

TABLE I LAMINA PROPRIA AND EPITHELIAL T CELL POPULATIONS IN NORMAL HUMAN INTESTINE.

Lamina Propria		**Epithelium**	
80%	CD4+ T cells	80%	CD8+ T cells
20%	CD8+ T cells	10%	CD4+ T cells
<1%	γ/δ TcR+ T cells	12%	CD3-, CD7+ non T cells
Few	VLA-1+ T cells	6%	CD3+,4-,8- T cells
		11%	γ/δ TcR+ T cells
		50%	VLA-1+
		44%	CD45R0+
		90%	HML-1+

INTESTINAL T CELL SUBPOPULATIONS IN DISEASE

It was originally hoped that immunohistochemistry would detect changes in mucosal T cell populations of relevance to the diagnosis and pathogenesis of disease. Mostly however this has not been the case. In ulcerative colitis, Crohn's disease and CD there are increased density of T cells within the lamina propria, however their phenotype is predominantly CD4 and any changes seen from controls are minor (4,7,15). Recently it has been shown that in Crohn's disease there are numerous CD25+ T cells in the lamina propria, whereas these cells are inconspicuous in ulcerative colitis and normal lamina propria (16). Activated lamina propria T cells are also seen in CD (17).

CHANGES IN IEL IN DISEASE:

T CELL SUBSET MARKERS

In inflammatory bowel disease there are no changes in the relative ratio of CD4 and CD8 cells in the epithelium (7,15). There is increased number of CD45R0+ IEL in both Crohn's and CD suggesting T cell activation in these conditions (3,11). The relative frequencies of CD3-,7+ IEL; CD3+,4-,8- IEL and those expressing the $\gamma\delta$ TcR in normal and diseased bowel have been the subject of recent interest. One of the main problems involved in determining if a change is specific for CD is the need for disease controls, i.e. patients with a flat mucosa and raised IEL densities but who are not gluten sensitive. The population of CD3-,7+ IEL is lost in CD, however it is also absent in patients with a flat mucosa who are gluten refractive (15), and in patients with a flat mucosa caused by tropical sprue (Spencer and Mac Donald, personal observation). Jenkins (18) was the first to suggest that there might be a population of subset negative T cells in the epithelium in CD. This was later confirmed by double staining (5). Importantly the increase in the relative proportion of CD3+,4-,8- T cells was only seen in CD and not in other diseases with flat mucosa (5) (Spencer, and MacDonald personal observation). The increase was also present in coeliacs with normal mucosal morphology on a gluten-free diet (5).

$\gamma\delta$ TCR EXPRESSION IN IEL

One of the most important recent advances in CD has been the observation that there is an increase in the frequency of $\gamma\delta$ TcR+ IEL in CD (14,19) which persists when the patient is on a gluten free diet (14) (E.Savilahti, personal communication). This increase is not seen in patients with a flat mucosa due to tropical sprue or in patients with cows milk protein intolerance (19,20). Thus it would appear to be a permanent difference in the epithelium of coeliac patients, which may even precede the development of overt disease. It is considered unlikely that $\gamma\delta$ TcR+ IEL play a primary role in the development of the flat mucosa since they are not abundant in diseases such as tropical sprue, where there is also villous atrophy (21). However they may be cytotoxic cells and be responsible for the surface enterocyte damage that is so striking in untreated CD (21).

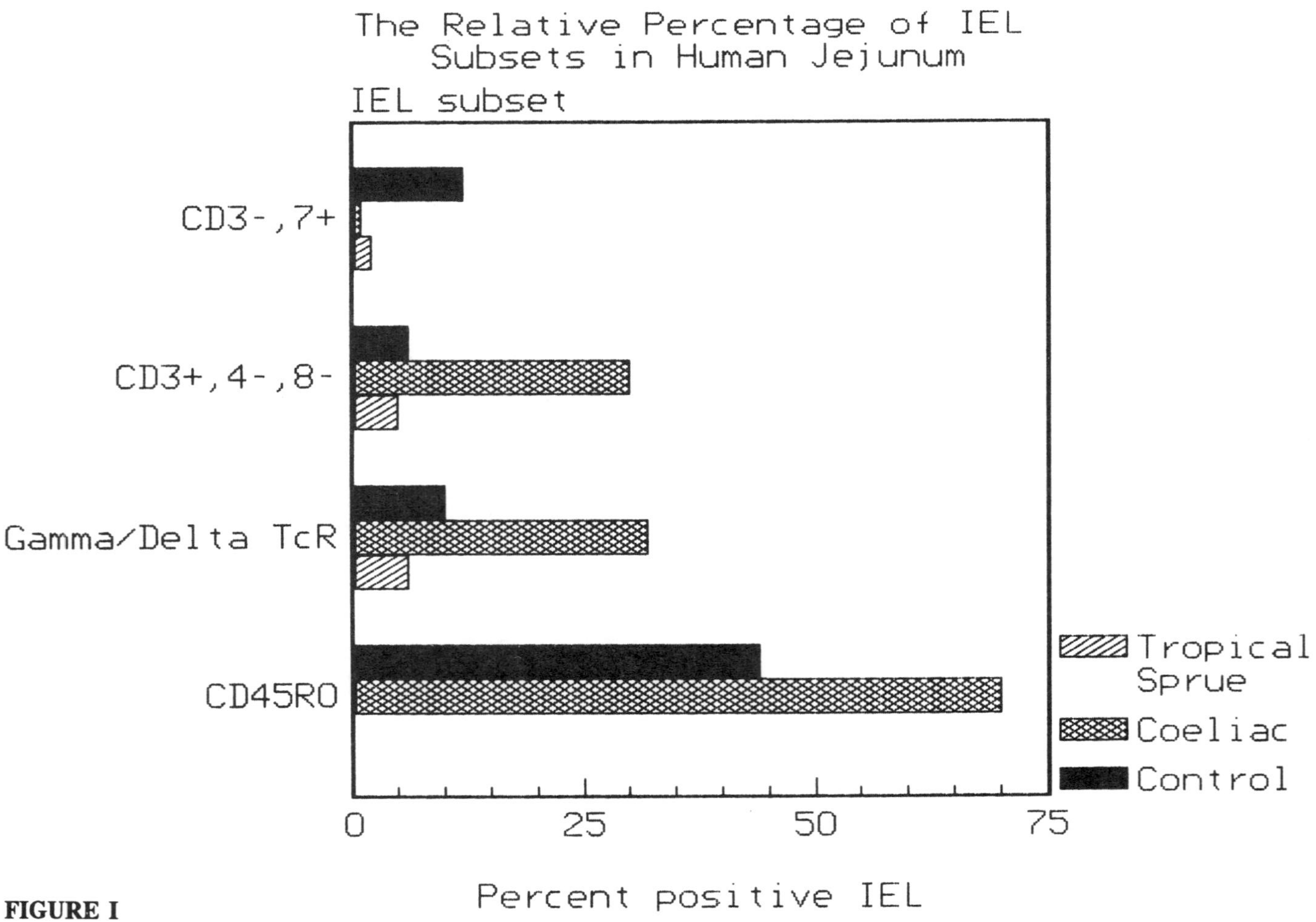
The Relative Percentage of IEL
Subsets in Human Jejunum
IEL subset
CD3-,7+
CD3+,4-,8-
Gamma/Delta TcR
CD45RO
0
25
50
75
Percent positive IEL
Tropical Sprue
Coeliac
Control

FIGURE I

The $\tau\delta$ TcR+ IEL in CD differ from those in the blood in that most of them are recognised by the monoclonal antibody δTCS-1, whereas these cells are few in blood. This antibody recognises T cells using Vδ1/Jδ1, with various Vτ genes (22). Until the recognition element of these T cells is established the significance of this observation will be unclear. A summary of the percentages of IEL subsets in normal and coeliac intestine and in tropical sprue are shown in Fig 1.

REFERENCES

1 Janossy G, Tidman N, Selby WS, Thomas JA, Granger S, Kung PC, and Goldstein G. Human T lymphocytes of inducer and suppressor type occupy different microenvironments. Nature 1980;288:81-84.

2 Malizia G, Trejdosiewicz LK, Wood GM, Howdle PD, Janossy G and Losowsky MS. The microenvironment in coeliac disease: T cell phenotypes and expression of the T2 "T blast" antigen by small bowel lymphocytes. Clin exp Immunol 1985;60:437-446.

3 Harvey J, Jones DB and Wright DH. Leucocyte common antigen expression on T cells in normal and inflamed human gut. Immunology 1989;68:13-17.

4 Kelly J, O'Farrelly C, O'Mahoney C, Weir DG and Feighery C. Immunoperoxidase demonstration of the cellular composition of the normal and coeliac small bowel. Clin exp Immunol 1987;68:177-188.

5 Spencer J, MacDonald TT, Diss TC, Walker-Smith JA, Ciclitira PJ and Isaacson PG. Changes in intraepithelial lymphocyte sub-populations in coeliac disease and enteropathy associated T cell lymphoma (malignant histiocytosis of the intestine). Gut 1989;30:339-346.

6 Spencer J, Dillon SB, Isaacson PG, and MacDonald TT. T cell subclasses in human fetal ileum. Clin Exp Immunol 1986;65:553.

7 Selby WS, Janossy G, Bofill M and Jewell DP. Intestinal lymphocyte subpopulations in inflammatory bowel disease: an analysis by immunohistological and cell isolation techniques. Gut 1984;25:32-40.

8 Jarry A, Cerf-Bensussan N, Brousse N, Selz F and Guy-Grand D. Subsets of CD3+ T cell receptor ($\alpha\beta$ or $\tau\delta$) and CD3- lymphocytes isolated from normal human gut epithelium display phenotypical features different from their counterparts in peripheral blood. Eur J Immunology 1990;20:1097-1104.

9 Cerf-Bensussan N, Jarry A, Brousse N, Lisowska-Grospierre B, Guy-Grand D and Griscelli C. A monoclonal antibody (HML-1) defining a novel membrane molecule present on human intestinal lymphocytes. Eur J Immunol 1987;17:1279-1285.

10 Choy MY, Richman PI, Horton ME and MacDonald TT. Expression of the VLA family of integrins in human intestine. J Pathology 1990;160:35-40.

11 Brandtzaeg P, Bosnes V, Halstensen TS, Scott H, Sollid LM and Valnes KN. T lymphocytes in human gut epithelium express preferentially the $\alpha\beta$ antigen receptor and are often CD45/UCHL1-positive. Scand J Immunology 1989;30:123-128.

12 Spencer J, Isaacson PG and MacDonald TT. Heterogeneity in intraepithelial lymphocyte subpopulations in fetal and post-natal human small intestine. J Pediatr Gastroenterol Nutr 1989;9:173-177.

13 Groh V, Porcelli S, Fabbi M, Lanier L, Picker LJ, Anderson T, Warnke RA, Bhan AK, Strominger JL and Brenner MB. Human lymphocytes bearing the T cell receptor $\tau\delta$ are phenotypically diverse and evenly distributed throughout the lymphoid system. J Exp Med 1989;169:1277-1294.

14 Halstensen TS, Scott H and Brandtzaeg P. Intraepithelial T cells of the TcR$\tau\delta$+ CD8- and Vδ1/Jδ1+ phenotypes are increased in coeliac disease. Scand J Gastroenterol 1989;30:665-672.

15 Hirata I, Berrebi G, Austin LL, Keren D and Dobbins WO. Immunohistological characterization of intraepithelial and lamina propria lymphocytes in control ileum and colon and in inflammatory bowel disease. Dig Dis Sciences 1986;31:593-603.

16 Choy MY, Walker-Smith JA, Williams CB, and MacDonald TT. Differential expression of CD25 on mucosal T cells and macrophages distinguishes the lesions in ulcerative colitis and Crohn's disease. Gut 1990 (in press).

17 MacDonald TT. The role of activated T lymphocytes in gastrointestinal disease. Clin Exp Allergy 1990;20:247-252.
18 Jenkins D, Goodall A and Scott BB. T-lymphocyte populations in normal and coeliac small intestinal mucosa defined by monoclonal antibodies. Gut 1986;27:1330-1337.
19 Spencer J, Isaacson PG, Diss TC and MacDonald TT. Expression of disulphide linked and non-disulphide linked forms of the T cell receptor gamma/delta heterodimer in human intestinal intraepithelial lymphocytes. Eur J Immunol 1989;19:1335-1339.
20 Spencer J, Isaacson PG, Diss TC and MacDonald TT. Subsets of gamma/ delta T cells in human intestinal epithelium. In: Advances in Mucosal Immunology. Thomas T MacDonald, Stephen J Challacombe et al. Kluwer Academic Press, Lancaster 1990;pp 57-60.
21 Viney J, Spencer J and MacDonald TT. Gamma/delta T cells in the gut epithelium. Gut 1990;31:841-844.
22 Borst J, Wicherink A, Van Dongen JJM, De Vries E et al. Non-random expression of T cell receptor γ and δ variable gene segments in functional T lymphocyte clones from human peripheral blood. Eur J Immunol 1989;19:1559-1568.

PERSISTENT INCREASE OF INTRA-EPITHELIAL T-CELL RECEPTOR τδ CELLS IN COELIAC DISEASE

Ph.M. Kluin, A.S. Peña, B.O. Roep, M.L. Mearin, G.J.A. Offerhaus, J.J. Schweizer, E.J. Dreef, F. Koning. Dept. of Pathology, Gastroenterology, Paediatrics and Immunohematology, University Medical Center, Leiden, The Netherlands.

Expression of the τ/δ T-cell receptor (TRCτδ) on intra-epithelial lymphocytes (IEL) in coeliac disease (CD) was studied by quantitative immunohistology of small intestinal biopsy specimens. Biopsies obtained from 3 CD patients with active disease, 5 patients on a gluten-free diet, 3 HLA-matched and 3 other controls were studied. Significantly more TRCτδ IEL were found in patients with active CD than in controls (TRCτδ/CD3: 0.47 versus 0.13, respectively). The increase persisted in 4 out of 5 patients on a gluten free diet (TRCτδ/CD3 ratio: 0.36), 3 patients being treated for more than 12 years. In all cases the increase was specifically found within the epithelium and not in the lamina propria. In contrast to blood TRCτδ T-cells, a relatively predominant usage of the Vδ-1 gene was suggested by a reactivity with the δ-TCS-1 monoclonal antibody. One of the proposed pathogenetic mechanisms in CD is a gluten dependent destruction of epithelial cells by IEL. In view of their possible role as constitutively cytolytic cells, our results suggest that TRCτδ-IEL are involved in the pathogenesis of CD.

INTRODUCTION

CD is characterized by gluten-dependent small intestinal villous atrophy. Presumably, in concert with a distinct genetic background, an immunological response leads to epithelial cell destruction (1-6). To clarify the mechanism, knowledge of the inflammatory cells within the affected intestine and especially of the intra-epithelial lymphocytes (IEL) will be of importance. In the normal mouse, most IEL as well as intra-epidermal cells express the τδ T-cell receptor (TCRτδ) (7-10).
These constitutively cytolytic cells may be important for maintenance of the epithelial integrity by selective killing of infected, transformed or damaged cells (11). This may correlate with the observations that TCRτδ cells can recognize heat shock proteins that are evolutionary conserved between bacteria and mammals (12-16). In contrast to the mouse, however, normal human IEL do not predominantly express the TCRτδ (17). In CD an increase of CD4- CD8- ("double negative") IEL (18) and more recently also increased numbers of TCRτδ IEL have been reported (19,20).
We confirm that in contrast to HLA-matched controls, high numbers of TCRτδ+ IEL are indeed present in active CD patients and that they persist during treatment with a gluten-free diet.

METHODS

<u>Coeliac disease patients and controls</u>: the diagnosis of CD was made according to the ESPGAN criteria (21). The study population comprised 3 patients with active CD, 5 CD patients on a gluten-free diet, 2 patients with suspicion of CD, 3 HLA-matched

M. L. Mearin and C. J. J. Mulder (eds.), Coeliac Disease, 57–64.

matched controls without CD and 3 other controls (Table I). From the patients with active disease, biopsies were taken at presentation of disease (n=1) and during a gluten provocation test after a gluten-free diet (n=2). The 5 treated patients were evaluated 3 months to > 30 years after withdrawal of gluten. One patient (case 1) was investigated both at presentation and 3 months after start of the diet. Two HLA-matched patients were suspected of CD but did not meet the ESPGAN-criteria: patient 8 had villous atrophy on a normal diet. After 3 years on a gluten free diet, the control intestinal biopsy was normal. At the moment she has been on a gluten containing diet for 2 years but she did not develop villous atrophy. Patient no 9 (no diet) was suspected of CD clinically. Repeated biopsies showed a slight increase of IEL and a minor degree of villous changes. A gluten provocation test was not performed. The HLA-matched controls included 2 mothers of CD patients with non-specific bowel complaints and normal histology of jejunal biopsies. Three children with complaints different from CD served as other controls (Table I).

TABLE I SURVEY OF PATIENTS

Case	Disease State	Age	Sex	Histology	HLA-Typing
Coeliac disease, active:					
1a	presentation	7	m	3	DR3/DQw2
2	gluten challenge	4	m	3	DR3/DR7/DQw2
3	gluten challenge	61	f	3	DR4/DR5
Coeliac disease, gluten free diet:					
1b	diet 3 months	7	m	1	DR3/DQw2
4	diet 18 months	45	f	1	DR3/DRw14/DQw2
5	diet 12 years	23	f	1	DR3/DR7/DQw2
6	diet 17 years	35	f	1	DR3/DR7/DQw2
7	diet > 30 years	68	f	2	DR3/DQw2
Suspected of coeliac disease:					
8	gluten challenge	8	f	0	DR3/DQw2
9	presentation	38	f	1	DR3/DR7/DQw2
Controls, HLA-matched:					
10	Mother CD	62	f	0	DR3/DQw2
11	Mother CD	46	f	0	DR5/DR7/DQw2
12	M. Crohn ileum	41	m	0	DR5/DR7/DQw2
Controls, others:					
13	Short stature	4	m	0	DRw8/DRw14/DQw1
14	Obstipation	4	m	0	DR5/DR9/DQw3/DQw7
15	Lactase deficiency	11	m	0	nd

0 = normal; 1 = minimal abnormalities; 2 = partial villous atrophy; 3 = subtotal villous atrophy; nd = not done; 1a/1b = same patients; CD = coeliac disease.

Jejunal biopsies were taken with a modified Rubin and Quinton instrument and were snap-frozen. Three step immunoperoxidase tests on 5 μm thick tissue sections consisted of a primary mouse-monoclonal antibody (MOAB), a second layer of rabbit-anti-mouse peroxidase-conjugated antiserum (Dakopatts, Copenhagen, Denmark) and a third layer of swine-anti-rabbit peroxidase-conjugated antiserum (Dakopatts). Staining was performed with 3-amino-9-ethylcarbazol. Slides were counterstained with Harris hematoxylin. Serial sections were stained by the following monoclonal MOABS: Leu-1 (CD5), Leu-2a (CD8), Leu-3a (CD4), Leu-4 (CD3) (all obtained from Becton Dickinson, Mountain View, CA), CLB-Tll (CD2; Central Laboratory of Blood Transfusion, Amsterdam, The Netherlands), WT-1 (CD7; Sanbio, Uden, The Netherlands) anti-TCR-βF1, abti-TCR-δ1 and δ-TCS-1 (T-cell Sciences, Cambridge, MA); δ-TCS-1 probably recognizes the Vδ1-protein (22). Anti-BB3 (probably recognizing the Vδ3-gene product [23,24]) was a generous gift of Dr. L. Moretta (INRC, Genova, Italy). anti-TiγA is a moab specific for the Vγ9-JγP-Cγ1-gene product (25) and was generously provided by Dr. T. Hercend (Villejuif, France).

Cell counts: in biopsy specimens without villous atrophy, cell counts were performed in the middle 3/4 segments of longitudinally sectioned villi. In biopsies with villous atrophy, surface areas were tested. Corresponding areas were counted in serial sections stained with different moabs. Immunoreactive IEL were counted per total number of cell nuclei (N-tot $\geq$ 200 in each biopsy; in the control biopsies of patients 13-15 with few IEL, 300-600 cells were counted). The total number of CD3+ IEL (N-CD3) per 100 epithelial cells (X) was calculated by:

$$X = 100 \times \text{N-CD3} / (\text{N-tot.} - \text{N-CD3}).$$

Since all TCR$\alpha\beta$ and TCR$\gamma\delta$ T-lymphocytes bear the CD3 molecule (25), numbers of TCR$\alpha\beta$ (Y) and TCR$\gamma\delta$ (Z) cells per 100 epithelial cells can be calculated by:

$$Y = 100 \times \text{N-TCR}\alpha\beta / (\text{N-tot.} - \text{N-CD3}).$$

$$Z = 100 \times \text{N-TCR}\gamma\delta / (\text{N-tot.} - \text{N-CD3}).$$

RESULTS

All small intestinal biopsy specimens of patients with active CD showed subtotal villous atrophy (Table I). Increased numbers of CD3+ IEL (as expressed per 100 epithelial cells) were present as compared with HLA-matched and other controls (Table II, Fig. 1). Using TCR-specific monoclonal antibodies, a relative increase of anti-TCR-δ1 (TCR$\gamma\delta$) cells over anti-TCR-βF1 (TCR$\alpha\beta$) cells was observed. In individual cases, the numbers of TCR$\gamma\delta$ plus TCR$\alpha\beta$ IEL were equivalent to the numbers of CD3 IEL. This is consistent with the finding that the CD3 molecule is structurally associated with either the TCR$\gamma\delta$ or TCR$\alpha\beta$ receptor (26), and allowed us to use the TCR$\gamma\delta$/CD3 ratio. This ratio increased from 0.10 $\pm$ 0.08 in 6 controls to 0.47 + 0.07 in 3 patients with active CD (significance of difference: $p<0.05$ by the Wilcoxon ranking test). No apparent increase of TCR$\gamma\delta$ cells within the lamina propria was observed. Five CD patients on a gluten free diet, three of them being treated for more than 12 years, were also studied. Four out of 5 biopsies showed minimal histological abnormalities (Table I). Except for patient 4, all biopsies contained increased numbers of TCRγδ IEL (TCRγδ/CD3 0.36 ± 0.17; $p<0.05$ as compared with controls; Table II, Fig. 1).

TABLE II IMMUNOPHENOTYPE OF INTRAEPITHELIAL LYMPHOCYTES

CASE	CD2	CD3	CD5	CD7	CD4	CD8	γδ	αβ	δTCS1	BB3	TiγA	γδ* CD3	γδ* αβ
	per 100 petihelial cells												
Coeliac disease, active:													
1a	72	94	41	88	0	55	35	56	23	0	2	0.37	0.63
2	-	198	73	174	1	57	106	58	76	21	16	0.54	1.83
3	57	60	24	61	1	58	30	42	16	0	2	0.50	0.71
Coeliac disease, diet:													
1b	14	24	12	23	1	13	11	15	11	2	0	0.46	0.73
4	27	34	13	33	0	23	3	28	4	0	0	0.09	0.11
5	54	48	-	47	0	24	18	38	9	1	0	0.38	0.47
6	28	44	21	51	1	20	26	25	13	0	3	0.59	1.04
7	62	61	23	63	3	52	18	51	11	5	2	0.30	0.35
Suspected of coeliac disease:													
8	23	24	-	29	0	23	6	20	1	0	0	0.24	0.30
9	29	42	18	44	4	30	18	22	4	0	4	0.43	0.82
Controls, HLA-matched:													
10	15	28	25	23	1	21	1	19	0	0	0	0.04	0.05
11	16	22	20	27	0	16	1	22	0	0	0	0.05	0.05
12	11	15	5	17	1	11	2	12	0	0	0	0.13	0.17
Controls, others:													
13	nd	9.1	nd	9.8	nd	nd	1.5	7.3	nd	nd	nd	0.16	0.21
14	nd	11.5	nd	13.6	nd	nd	2.6	9.0	nd	nd	nd	0.23	0.29
15	nd	13.9	nd	14.3	nd	nd	0.0	11.4	nd	nd	nd	0.00	0.00

IEL = intraepithelial lymphocytes; γδ = TCRγδ; - = staining too weak; nd = not done; αβ = TCRαβ; 1a = patients S at presentation; 1b = same patient, 3 months after start of gluten free diet; * number of TCRγδ per number of CD3 cells or per number of TCRαβ cells.

The 2 patients who clinically were suspected of CD had no (Case 8) or minimal (case 9) histological abnormalities. However, the TCRγδ/CD3 ratios were abnormal (0.24 and 0.43, respectively; Table II, Fig. 1). To investigate expression of Vγ and Vδ genes by TCRγδ IEL, we tested TCRγδ IEL with monoclonal antibodies, normally recognizing 2 complementary TCRγδ T-cell subsets in the peripheral blood. As shown in Table 2, a majority of TCRγδ IEL was δ-TCS-1 positive in CD patients. In control biopsies, their numbers were too low for reliable immunohistological quantitation. The 2 patients suspected of CD (cases 8 and 9) without villous atrophy, had increased numbers of TCR$\gamma\delta$ IEL, but no apparent increase of δ-TCS-1 cells. In these patients, but also in others (Table II), the numbers of δ-TCS-1 plus BB3 and TiγA cells was lower than the number of anti-TCR-δ1 cells, suggesting that cells with expression of other TCR$\gamma\delta$-genes may be present.

FIGURE I

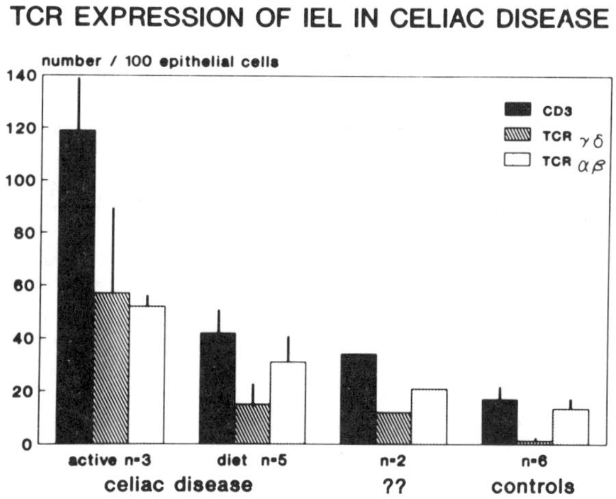

(Numbers are expresed per 100 epithelial cells. IEL are marked by monoclonal antibodies reactive with the TCR$\alpha\beta$, TCR$\gamma\delta$ and CD3 antigens. Vertical lines indicate standard desviation.; ?? = 2 patients suspected of coeliac disease.)

Immunohistological analysis of other T-cell related antigens in CD showed that IEL consistently were CD7 positive and CD4 negative (Table II). In the majority of the CD cases, the number of CD8 positive cells paralleled the number of TCR$\alpha\beta$ cells. Although co-expression of CD8 in the TCR$\alpha\beta$ and TCR$\gamma\delta$ subsets is impossible to determine definitively without performing double labelling, cell counts indicated the apparent expression of CD8 on a part of the TCR$\gamma\delta$ cells in case 3.

DISCUSSION

The small intestinal epithelium of patients with CD contains increased numbers of intra-epithelial T cells with expression of the $\gamma\delta$ T cell receptor (TCR$\gamma\delta$). This is in contrast to the lamina propia where relatively very low numbers were invariably present, both in controls and CD. The numbers of TCR$\gamma\delta$ positive IEL in controls were similar for the HLA-matched family members of CD patients and other cases. Therefore, our data indicate that not the genetic predisposition, nor a site-specific distribution, but most likely the disease itself is associated with an increase of TCR$\gamma\delta$ IEL. The results in the controls correspond with the data reported in the literature, demonstrating that equally low percentages of TCR$\gamma\delta$cells are present in the human gut and in peripheal blood (17). Thus, the normal situation in man is different from the mouse, where intra-epithelial cells of the skin and gut preferen-

tially express the TCRγδ (7-10). The increase of TCRγδ IEL persisted with treatment in most patients even after restoration of the normal villous architecture. Notably, high numbers of TCRγδ persisted in 3 patients treated with a gluten-free diet from more than 12 years. Most likely, these cells are maintained by a low but continuous exposure to gliadin during treatment, since a completely gluten free diet is rarely if ever achieved.
Our data demonstrate that TCRγδ IEL in CD preferentially use the Vδ1 gene segment. Preliminay data obtained from flow cytometry of isolated and in vitro cultured IEL also suggested a predominant δ-TCS-1 expression in CD: in 2 patients studied, 97% and 60% of all TCRγδ+ cells were δ-TCS-1 positive after 3 weeks of culture; 3% and 29% were BB3/TiγA positive, respectively (F.Koning unpublished observation). This is in contrast with blood TCRγδ+ cells which mainly are BB3/TiγA positive (22-25) (preliminary data in controls and in 6 CD patients; F. Koning unpublished observation). However, this preferential expression of Vδ1 by IEL is not necessarily disease-related since strong site-specific and age-related differences in usages of Vγ chain segments have been reported (8,27). As a consequence and as recently suggested (20), the increase of δ-TCS-1 cells in CD may reflect expansion of resident TCRγδ, δ-TCS-1 positive cells resulting from antigenic exposure. To get more insight in the usage of different V-genes by IEL, however, analysis of large series of biopsies obtained from controls and patients at different ages and with different diseases is necessary.

The function of TCRγδ cells is largely unknown. Their preferential presence within mouse epithelia has prompted the hypothesis that these cells represent an immunological barrier against foreign antigens. TCRγδ cells, like TCRαβ cells, might recognize small peptides in association with MHC or MHC-like molecules (11, 26). Evidence has been presented for a specific recognition of mycobacterial antigens or heat shock proteins (12-16). In CD, specific IEL (either TCRαβ or TCRγδ cells) might recognize epithelial cells altered by gliadin. Perhaps, recognition is triggered by a primary adenoviral infection, leading to cross reacting gliadin-specific T-cells (29). Cytolytic TCRγδ IEL cells might be activated and accumulate either by direct antigenic stimulation (gliadin), or indirectly by exposure to heat shock proteins released from otherwise damaged epithelial cells (27). Probably, due to a continuing but low exposure to gliadin during treatment, TCRγδ IEL will persist and may be implicated in the renewed epithelial cell destruction after re-exposure to higher doses of gliadin. Our findings suggest that assessment of the number of TCRγδ IEL may be an additional diagnostic tool in CD. Further studies are necessary to determine whether the increase is specific for CD or can be found in other diseases associated with villous atrophy like tropical sprue and cow milk allergy as well, and whether this assay can be used as an additional diagnostic test for CD. Moreover, in vitro tests of cloned TCRγδ IEL, successfully isolated from several CD patients, are in progress to elucidate their possible function in the pathogenesis of this disease.

REFERENCES

1 Strober W. Gluten-sensitive enteropathy. An abnormal Immunologic response of the gastrointestinal tract to a dietary protein. In: Shorter RG, Kirsne JB eds. Gastrointestinal

immunity for the clinician. New York: Grune and Stratton Inc.: 1985;75-112.
2 Keuning JJ, Peña AS, van Hooff JP, van Leeuwen A, van Rood JJ. HLA-Dw3 associated with coeliac disease. Lancet 1976;i:506-8.
3 Mearin ML, Biemond I, Peña AS, Polanco I, Vazquez I, Schreuder GThM, de Vries RRP, van Rood JJ. HLA-DR phenotypes in Spanish coeliac children: their contribution to the understanding of the disease. Gut 1983;24:532-7.
4 Tosi R, Vismara D, Tanigaki N, Ferrara GB, Cicimara F, Buffalana W, Folle D, Auricchio S. Evidence that coeliac disease is primarily associated with a DC locus allelic specificity. Clin Immunol Immunopath 1983;8:395-404.
5 Roep BO, Bontrop RE, Peña AS, van Eggermont MCJA, van Rood JJ, Giphart MJ. An HLA-DQ alpha allele identified at DNA and protein level is strongly associated with coeliac disease. Human Immunology 1988;23:271-9.
6 Sollid LM, Markussen G, Ek J, Gjerde H, Vartdal F, Thorsby E. Evidence for a primary association of coeliac disease to a particular HLA-DQα/β heterodimer. J Exp Med 1989;169:345-50.
7 Goodman Th, Lefrancois L. Expression of the τ-δ T-cell receptor on intestinal CD8+ intraepithelial lymphocytes. Nature 1988;333:855-8.
8 Bonneville M, Janeway ChA, Ito K, Haser W, Ishida I, Nakanishi N, Tonegawa S. Intestinal intraepithelial lymphocytes are a distinct set of τδ T Cells. Nature 1988;346:479-81.
9 Koning F, Stingl G, Yokahama WM, Yamada H, Lee Maloy W, Tschachler E, Shevach ES, Coligan JE. Identification of a T3-associated τδ T cell receptor on Thy-1+ dendritic epidermal cell lines. Science 1987;236:834-7.
10 Kuziel WA, Takashima A, Bonyhadi M, Bergstresser PR, Allison JP, Tigelaar RE, Tucker PW. Regulation of T-cell receptor τ-chain RNA expression in murine Thy-1+ dendritic epidermal cells. Nature 1987;328:263-6.
11 Janeway ChA, Jones B, Hayday A. Specificity and function of T cells bearing τδ receptors. Immunol Today 1988;9:73-6.
12 O'Brien RL, Happ MP, Dallas A, Palmer E, Kubo R, Born WK. Stimulation of a major subset of lymphocytes expressing Tcell receptor τδ by an antigen derived from mycobacterium tuberculosis. Cell 1989;57:667-74.
13 Janis EM, Kaufman SHE, Schwartz RH, Padoll DM. Activation of τδ T cells in the primary immune respons to mycobacterium tuberculosis. Science 1989;244:713-6.
14 Holoshitz J, Koning F, Coligan JE, de Bruyn J, Strober S. Isolation of CD4- CD8- mycobacteria-reactive T lymphocyte clones from rheumatoid arthritis synovial fluid. Nature 1989;339:226-30.
15 Modlin RL, Pirmez C, Hofman FM, Torigian V, Uyemura K, Rea ThH, Bloom BR, Brenner MB. Lymphocytes bearing specific τδ T-cell receptors in human infectious disease lesions. Nature 1989;339:544-8.
16 Raulet DH. Antigens for τ/δ T cells. Nature 1989;339:342-3.
17 Groh V, Porcelli S, Fabbi M, Lanier LL, Picker LJ, Anderson T, Warnke RA, Bhan AK, Strominger JL, Brenner MB. Human lymphocytes bearing T cell receptor τ/δ are phenotypically diverse and evenly distributed throughout the lymphoïd system. J Exp Med 1989;169:1277-94.
18 Spencer JO, MacDonald TT, Diss TC, Walker-Smith JA, Ciclitira PJ, Isaacson PG. Changes in intraepithelial lymphocyte subpopulations in coeliac disease and enteropathy associated T cell lymphoma (malignant histiocytosis of the intestine). Gut 1989;30:339-46.
19 Hastensen TS, Scott H, Brandtzaeg P. Intraepithelial T cells of the TcRτ/δ+ CD8- and Vδ1/Jδ1+ phenotypes are increased in coeliac disease. Scan J Immunol 1989;30:665-672.
20 Spencer J, Isaacson PG, Diss T, MacDonald TT. Expression of disulphide-linked and non-disulphide linked forms of the T cell receptor τ/δ heterodimer in human intestinal intraepithelial lymphocytes. Eur J Immunol 1989;19-1335-8.
21 Meeuwisse GW. Diagnostic criteria in coeliac disease. Acta Paediatr Scand 1970;59:461-3.
22 Lanier LL, Ruitenberg J, Bolhuis RLH, Borst J, Phillips JH, Testi R. Structural and serological heterogeneity of τ/δ T cell antigen receptor expression in thymus and peripheal blood. Eur J Immunol 1988;18:1985-92.
23 Bottino C, Tambussi G, Ferrini S, Ciccone E, Varese P, Mingari MC, Moretta L, Moretta A.

Two subsets of human T lymphocytes expressing τ/δ antigen receptor are identifiable by monoclonal antibodies directed to two distinct molecular forms of the receptor. J Exp Med 1988;168:491-505.
24 Triebel F, Faure F, Mami-Chouaib F, Jitsukawa S, Griscelli A, Genevee C, Roman-Roman S, Hercend T. A novel Vδ gene expressed predominantly in the TiτA fraction of τ/δ+ peripheal lymphocytes. Eur J Immunol 1988;18:2021-7.
25 Triebel F, Faure F, Graziani M, Jitsukawa S, Lefranc M-P, Hercend T. A unique V-J-C-rearranged gene encodes a τ protein expressed on the majority of CD3+ T cell receptor -α/β-circulating lymphocytes. J Exp Med 1988;167:694-99.
26 Davis MM, Bjorkman PM. T-cell antigen receptor genes and T-cell recognition. Nature 1988;334:395-402.
27 Asarnow DM, Kuziel WA, Bonyhadi M, Tigelaar E, Tucker PW, Allison JP. Limited diversity of $\tau\delta$ antigen receptor genes of Thy-1+ dendritic epidermal cells. Cell 1988;55:837-47.
28 Kagnoff MF, Austin RK, Hubert JJ, Bernadin JE, Kasarda DD. Possible role for a human adenovirus in the pathogenesis of coeliac disease. J Exp Med 1984;160:1544-57.
29 Karagiannis JA, Priddle JD, Jewell DP. Cell-mediated immunity to a synthetic gliadin peptide resembling a sequence from adenovirus 12. The Lancet 1987;i:884-6.

T-CELL SUBPOPULATIONS IN COELIAC DISEASE; LONGTERM FOLLOW UP WITH A GLUTEN CONTAINING DIET.

T. Kutlu, N. Cerf-Bensussan, C. Rambau, N. Brousse and J. Schmitz. Dep. Paed., Inserm U132, Dep. Histopathol., Hôpital des Enfants Malades, Paris.

INTRODUCTION

The striking increase of T cells in the jejunal epithelium of patients with coeliac disease (CD) (1, 2, 3) suggests that intraepithelial lymphocytes (IEL) play a role in the constitution of crypt hyperplasia and villous atrophy. IEL might also be involved in the development of tolerance to gluten in some children whose intestinal lesions disappear despite gluten ingestion (4, 5). An important link in the chain of events leading to lymphocyte activation is the T-cell receptor (TCR) by which T cells recognize antigens. Previous studies have shown that a small fraction of IEL, with the TCR $\gamma/\delta+$, CD4- CD8- phenotype and using $V\delta 1/J\delta 1$ gene segment, is increased in CD (6-9). In order to get a better insight into the role of these cells in the development, the persistance and possibly also in the disappearance of intestinal lesions in CD, we decided to study the phenotypes of IEL, with special emphasis on their TCR, in children at different periods of their disease, and particularly after years on a gluten containing diet.

PATIENTS AND CONTROLS

Twenty one patients from 1 to 37 years of age were studied. Two of them (1 and 8 years of age) were studied at the time of diagnosis (Gr 1). Both had a typical malabsorption syndrome with failure to thrive and a flat mucosa. Six were strictly following a gluten free diet for 1 to 11 years. Their mucosa was normal (4 times) or showed moderate villous atrophy (V/C ratio > 1). Gluten challenge has not yet been performed in this group of children (Gr 2). The remaining 13 patients had confirmed CD according to ESPGAN criteria (10). Their diet contained gluten for 1 to 3 years (Gr 3, n=4), for 5 to 8 years (Gr 4, n=5) or more than 10 years (Gr 5, n=4). Severe villous atrophy (VA) was present in all cases in Gr 3 and 4, and in only 1 case out of 4 in Gr 5. In the other 3 cases of Gr 5 (transient CD) the duodenal mucosa was histologically normal in one patient (reported 10 years ago (4)) or showed slight VA (V/C ratio > 2) in the other 2 patients.
Control biopsies were obtained from adults undergoing intestinal surgery for gastric cancer or chronic pancreatitis (n=15) and from children with short stature (n=10).

METHODS

All biopsies were done with a paediatric Crosby capsule and were immediately frozen. Cryostat sections were stained by an immunoperoxidase technique (11) using monoclonal antibodies directed to CD3, CD4, CD8 CD25, HLA DR non polymorphic determinants (Becton Dickinson) and to the framework of TCR $\alpha\beta$ and TCR $\gamma\delta$ (βF1 and TCR δ1 respectively, gifts from Dr. M. Brenner). The subsets of TCR

M. L. Mearin and C. J. J. Mulder (eds.), Coeliac Disease, 65–70.

$\gamma\delta$+ cells were studied using monoclonal antibodies Ti γA, anti Ti Vδ2 (gifts from Dr. T. Hercend), δTCS1 (T cell Sciences) which react with TCR $\gamma\delta$+ cells using Vγ9, Vδ2, Vδ1/Jδ1 segments, respectively (12). The number of IEL stained with a given monoclonal antibody was estimated by counting the peroxidase-stained cells in the surface epithelium per 100 enterocytes (surface enterocytes = SE), 500 to 1000 enterocytes being counted for each monoclonal antibody.

RESULTS

Subpopulations of T cells in the surface epithelium are presented in the Table according to the stage of the disease when the biopsy was performed. The number of CD3+ IEL per 100 SE was significantly higher at the time of diagnosis than in age-matched controls ($p<0.05$). It decreased following gluten exclusion and recovery to a normal villous architecture, although not significantly ($p>0.05$) and reincreased markedly after reintroduction of gluten in the diet and reappearance of a flat mucosa ($p<0.05$). As time with a normal diet elapsed, numbers of CD3+ IEL decreased compared with those observed in patients of Gr. 3. The difference became significant ($p<0.05$) after 10 years.
The number of TCR $\alpha\beta$+ cells (as revealed by βF1 mab) showed parallel but even more significant variations. Their number was elevated at the time of diagnosis compared to pediatric controls ($p<0.01$). It decreased significantly ($p<0.01$) after exclusion of gluten and recovery of a normal villous architecture and reincreased markedly after reintroduction of gluten and reappearance of subtotal VA (STVA) ($p<0.01$). After 5 to 8 years of a normal diet, the numbers of βF1+ cells tended to decrease but the difference with patients from Gr. 3 was not significant; the decrease became significant after more than 10 years of a gluten containing diet for the 3 patients having recovered to a normal villous architecture (transient CD) ($p<0.01$). In the latter adult patients, the number of βF1+ IEL was not significantly different from that observed in adult controls. Most TCR $\alpha\beta$+ IEL were CD8+. Accordingly, variations of CD8+ IEL followed closely that of TCR $\alpha\beta$+ IEL. However, a moderate but significant increase in the numbers of CD4+ IEL was also observed in CD patients with a normal diet and STVA (3.4 ± 1.6) compared to patients without VA (1.6 ± 0.8) and to pediatric controls (2.0 ± 1.0) ($p<0.01$).
Numbers of TCR $\gamma\delta$+ IEL (TCR δ1+) per 100 SE, although very variable, were significantly higher in CD than in controls ($p<0.01$). In contrast to TCR $\alpha\beta$+ IEL, TCR $\gamma\delta$+ IEL did not vary significantly in numbers according to the diet or to the degree of villous atrophy. The numbers of TCR $\gamma\delta$+ IEL recognized by antibodies directed to Vδ2 and Vγ9 were comparable as expected since both antibodies usually detect overlapping subsets (12). Vδ2/Vγ9 IEL were moderately increased in CD but the difference was not significant. In contrast, a significant increase in the number of IEL using Vδ1/Jδ1 was observed ($p<0.05$). In addition, comparison of the numbers of IEL that stained with TCR δ1, δ TCS1, anti-TiVδ 2 and Ti γA monoclonal antibodies suggested that, in CD, a significant number of TCR $\gamma\delta$+ IEL expressed neither Vδ1/Jδ1 nor Vδ2/Vγ9 (6.3 ± 4.8) in contrast to normal TCR $\gamma\delta$+ IEL (controls 0.65 ± 0.65 and 13) or peripheral blood lymphocytes (12) ($p<0.01$). Finally, by comparing the mean of TCR δ1+ IEL (18.6 ± 11.6) and the mean of [(βF1 +

TCR 1+) - (CD4+ + CD8+)] IEL (14.4 ± 11.7), it was possible to deduce that approximately 75% of TCR $\gamma\delta$+ IEL were CD4- CD8- in CD.

Finally, signs of intestinal mononuclear cell activation varied with the stage of the disease. In all CD patients on a gluten-containing diet and with STVA (including 3 patients with STVA after 15 years on a normal diet, who were not considered in this study because of the poor preservation of the tissues preventing the count of IEL), numerous CD25+ cells were observed in the subepithelial lamina propria. Two patients had a small number of CD25+ IEL. HLA-DR antigens were strongly expressed by both surface and crypt enterocytes. This contrasted with findings in controls, in patients on a gluten-free diet or in transient CD. In all these cases, CD25+ cells were absent. HLA-DR expression was weak or absent on the crypt enterocytes except in one adult with transient CD in whom HLA-DR expression on the crypts remained elevated.

TABLE I T CELL SUBPOPULATIONS IN THE SURFACE EPITHELIUM OF COELIAC PATIENTS AND CONTROLS

	CD3	CD8	CD4	βF1	TCRδ1	Vγ9	Vδ2	δTCS1
Group 1:								
Active disease	57*	45	5	40	6	2	0.5	2
(n=2)	(54-60)#	(45-45)	(2-7)	(42-38)	(6-7)	(1-2)	(0.5-)	(2-2)
Group 2:								
Gluten free diet	44	21	1	20	21	3	3	10
(n=6)	(17)+	(3)	(0.5)	(6)	(16)	(3)	(2)	(8)
Gluten containing diet								
Group 3:								
. 1 to 3 years (n=4)	74	55	3	50	17	4	3	6
	(17)	(7)	(1)	(7)	(7)	(3)	(1)	(4)
Group 4:								
. 5 to 8 years (n=5)	63	44	3	36	22	5	5	7
	(21)	(13)	(1)	(12)	(13)	(2)	(2)	(6)
Group 5:								
. > 10 years								
- flat mucosa (n=1)	44	30	5	35	11	3	3	3
- transient CD (n=3)	43	21	2	21	21	4	4	10
	(8)	(7)	(1)	(5)	(8)	(0.5)	(0.5)	(3)
Controls:								
. children (n=10)	16	17	2	14	2	1	1	1
	(8)	(9)	(1)	(7)	(1)	(1)	(0.5)	(0.5)
. adults (n=15)	22	17	3	17	4	2	2	2
	(9)	(10)	(1)	(8)	(3)	(2)	(3)	(2)

* mean number of + IEL/100 enterocytes; # individual values; + standard deviation.

DISCUSSION

The mechanism by which gluten induces villous atrophy in CD is unknown but a large number of studies has emphasized the possible role of abnormally activated IEL (14). Recently, a small subset of CD4- CD8- TCR γδ-bearing IEL was found to be increased in coeliac patients, but not in tropical sprue (7) or in intractable diarrhoea of infancy with VA (15), suggesting that these cells may be of particular importance in the pathogenesis of CD. Our own observations confirmed the marked increase in the numbers of TCRγδ bearing IEL in CD either untreated or treated. In addition, we showed that this increase persisted in 3 patients having recovered a normal villous architecture in spite of a normal diet (transient CD). As previously observed (7, 8), the increase in TCR γδ+ IEL interested a subset of CD4- CD8- IEL using the Vδ1/Jδ1 segment. In addition, as also observed by Spencer (7), a significant number of TCR γδ+ IEL apparently using neither Vγ9/Vδ2 nor Vδ1/Jδ1 was observed in our CD patients. In contrast, such cells appear to be rare or absent in peripheral blood (12) as well as in normal intestinal epithelium (7, 13 and herein). Although this finding should be confirmed by double-labeling experiments, it may indicate the presence of a third subset of TCR γδ+ IEL in CD. Altogether, these observations suggest that some subsets of TCR γδ+ IEL are involved in the development of CD. However, the lack of variations according to the stage of the disease also indicates that these cells are not directly responsible for the villous atrophy. The functions of TCR γδ+ T cells (which represent less than 5% of peripheral T cells) are not yet well defined. Most studies have emphasized their cytotoxic properties, either MHC or non-MHC restricted (16). More recently, TCR γδ+ cells responsive to exogenous antigens, presented or not by autologous macrophages, were observed (17). Two recent observations regarding the possible role of TCR γδ+ cells may be more relevant to CD. On one hand, it has been shown that antigen-specific TCR γδ+ cells from nude mice, when injected in normal mice, were able to abrogate oral tolerance (18). On the other hand, a study of local cutaneous graft-versus-host reaction in mice has shown that after recovery, there was a prolonged local resistance to reinduction of epidermal lesions, possibly confered by Thyl+ TCR γδ+ epidermal cells (19). Further studies are therefore needed to understand whether TCR γδ+ cells are deleterious or not in CD.
In contrast, our study provides evidence that TCR αβ+ IEL are responsive to gluten and may play a role in the mechanism of the VA. Thus, TCR αβ+, mainly CD8+, IEL were elevated in patients on a normal diet and with STVA and markedly decreased after recovery of a normal villous architecture either after gluten exclusion or in the 3 patients with transient CD. Furthermore, presence of activated CD25+ mononuclear cells and high enterocytic HLA-DR expression reflecting the increased local secretion of lymphokines (20-22) correlated with the presence of increased numbers of TCR αβ+ and of villous atrophy. The mechanism by which TCR αβ+ cells might induce VA in CD remains to be elucidated. Studies of mouse graft-versus-host disease (23) where infiltrating T cells are TCR αβ+ lymphocytes (24) and of T cell-induced damage in human fetal organ culture (25), suggest that they may act either through the secretion of lymphokines or by being cytotoxic.
Finally, the long term evolution of the intestinal lesions and of the IEL subsets in a

group of coeliac patients left on a clinically well tolerated gluten-containing diet is striking. All these patients had subtotal villous atrophy one to three years after gluten reintroduction. The villous atrophy persisted unchanged except in 3 patients where it disappeared (once) or nearly so (twice) after more than 10 years. In contrast with the number of TCR $\tau\delta$+ IEL/100 SE which did not fluctuate with time, the number of TCR $\alpha\beta$+ IEL tended to decrease as time passed with a gluten containing diet. Although not significant from Gr. 4 to Gr. 3, the decrease was significant after 10 years from Gr. 5 to Gr. 3, numbers of CD8+, and of TCR $\alpha\beta$+ IEL falling in normal ranges. It thus seems that, at least in a subgroup of CD patients, progressive appearance of clonal anergy and tolerance to gluten is possible. Further studies may help to understand the relationship between the elevated level of TCR $\tau\delta$+ IEL, the probable abnormal reactivity of TCR $\alpha\beta$+ IEL to gluten and the strong association of CD with an HLA class II DQw2 heterodimer (26) and their respective contribution to the development of the disease as well as, in some patients, to epithelial recovery and to establishment of tolerance to gluten.

REFERENCES

1 Ferguson A, Murray D. Quantitation of human intraepithelial lymphocytes in human jejunum. Gut 1971;12:988.

2 Selby WS, Janossy G, Bofill M, Jewel DP. Lymphocyte subpopulations in the human small intestine. The findings in normal mucosa and in the mucosa of patients with adult coeliac disease. Clin Exp Immunol 1983;52:219.

3 Leigh RJ, Marsh MN, Crowe P, Kelly C, Garner V, Gordon D. Studies of intestinal lymphoid tissue. IX. Dose-dependent gluten-induced lymphoid infiltration of coeliac jejunal epithelium. Scand J Gastroenterol 1985;20:715.

4 Schmitz J, Jos J, Rey J. Transient mucosal atrophy in confirmed coeliac disease. In "Perspectives in Coeliac Disease", McNicholl B, McCarthy CF, Fottrell PF eds, Lancaster, MTP Press, 1978;259.

5 Schmitz J, Arnaud-Battandier F, Jos J. Rey J. Long term follow-up of childhood coeliac disease. Is there a natural recovery? Pediatr Res 1984;18:1054 (abstract).

6 Spencer J, McDonald TT, Diss TC, Walker-Smith JA, Ciclitira PJ, Isaacson PG. Changes in intraepithelial lymphocyte subpopulations in coeliac disease and enteropathy associated T-cell lymphoma (malignant histiocytosis of the intestine). Gut 1989;30:339.

7 Spencer J, Isaacson PG, Diss TC, McDonald TT. Expression of disulfide-linked and non-disulfide-linked forms of the T cell receptor τ/δ heterodimer in human intestinal intraepithelial lymphocytes. Eur J Immunol 1989;19:1335.

8 Halstensen TS, Scott H, Brandtzaeg P. Intraepithelial T cells of the TCR τ/δ+ CD8- and Vδ1/Jδ1+ phenotypes are increased in coeliac disease. Scand J immunol 1989;30:665.

9 Verkasalo MA, Arato A, Savilahti E, Tainio VM. Effect of diet and age on jejunal and circulating lymphocyte subsets in children with coeliac disease: persistence of CD4- CD8- intraepithelial T cells through treatment. Gut 1990;31:422.

10 Weijers HA, Lindquist B, Anderson CM, Rey J, Shmerling DH, Visakorpi JK, Hadorn B, Gruttner R. Round table discussion. Diagnosic; criteria in coeliac disease. Acta Paediatr Scand 1970;59:461.

11 Cerf-Bensussan N, Jarry A, Brousse N, Lisowska-Grospierre B, Guy-Grand D, Griscelli C. A monoclonal antibody (HML-1) defining a novel membrane molecule present on human intestinal lymphocytes. Eur J Immunol 1987;17:1279.

12 Miossec C, Faure F, Ferradini L, Roman-Roman S, Jitsukawa S, Ferrini S, Moretta A, Triebel F, Hercend T. Further analysis of the T cell receptor $\tau\delta$+ peripheral lymphocyte subset. The Vδ1 segment is expressed with either Cτ or Cα. J Exp Med 1990;171:1171.

13 Jarry A, Cerf-Bensussan N, Selz F, Brousse N, Guy-Grand D. Subsets of CD3+ (TCR $\alpha\beta$ or $\tau\delta$) and CD3- lymphocytes isolated from normal gut epithelium display phenotypical features

different from their counterparts in peripheral blood. Eur J Immunol 1990;20:1097.
14 Brantzaeg P, Halstensen TS, Kett K, Krajci P, Kvale D, Rogrum O, Scott H, Sollid LM. Immunobiology and immunopathology of human gut mucosa: humoral immunity and intraepithelial lymphocytes. Gastroenterology 1989;97:1562.
15 Cuenod B, Brousse N, Goulet O, De Potter S, Mougenot JF, Ricour C, Guy-Grand D, Cerf-Bensussan N. Classification of intractable diarrhoea in infancy using clinical and immunohistological criteria. Gastroenterology 1990;99:1037.
16 Raulet DH. The structure, function and molecular genetics of the T cell receptor. Ann Rev Immunol 1989;7:175.
17 Born W, Happ HP, Dallas A, Reardon C, Kubo R, Schinnick T, Brennan P, O'Brien R. Recognition of heat-shock proteins and cell function. Immunol Today 1990;11:40.
18 Fujihashi K, Kyono H, Aicker W, Green D, Singh B, Eldridge JH, McGhee JR. Immunoregulatory function of CD3+, CD4-, CD8-, T cells. T cell receptor positive T cells from nude mice abrogate oral tolerance. J Immunol 1989;143:3415.
19 Shiohara T, Moriya N, Gotoh C, Hayakawa J, Nagashima M, Saizawa K, Ishikawa H. Loss of epidermal integrity by T cell-mediated attack induces long-term local resistance to subsequent attack. I. Induction of resistance correlates with increase in thy 1+ epidermal cell numbers. J Exp Med 1990;171:1027.
20 Cerf-Bensussan N, Quaroni A, Kurnick JT, Bhan AK. Intraepithelial lymphocytes modulate Ia expression by intestinal epithelial cells. J Immunol 1984;132:2244.
21 Arnaud-Battandier F, Cerf-Bensussan N, Amsellen R, Schmitz J. Increased HLA-DR expression by enterocytes in children with coeliac disease. Gastroenterology 1986;91:1206.
22 Steiniger B, Falk P, Lohmuller M, van der Meide PH. Class II MHC antigens in the rat digestive system. Normal distribution and induced expression after interferon gamma treatment in vivo. Immunology 1989;68:507.
23 Guy-Grand D, Vassalli P. Gut injury in mouse graft-versus-host reaction. Study of its occurrence and mechanisms. J Clin Invest 1986;77:1584.
24 Guy-Grand D, Cerf-Bensussan N, Malissen B, Malassis-Seris M, Briottet C, Vassalli P. Two gut intraepithelial CD8+ lymphocyte populations with different T cell receptors: A role for the gut epithelium in T cell differentiation. J Exp Med: in press.
25 McDonald TT, Spencer J. Evidence tht activated mucosal T cells play a role in the pathogenesis of enteropathy in human small intestine. J Exp Med 1988;167:1341.
26 Sollid LM, Markussen G, Ek J, Gjerd H, Vartdal F, Thorsby E. Evidence for a primary association of coeliac disease to a particular HLA-DQ β heterodimer. J Exp Med 1989;169:345.

INTRAEPITHELIAL T-CELLS OF THE TcRτ/δ+CD8- AND Vδ1+ PHENOTYPES ARE STRIKINGLY INCREASED IN COELIAC DISEASE.

T.S. Halstensen, H. Scott, P. Brandtzaeg. Lab. Immunohistochemistry and Immunopathology (LIIPAT), Department of Pathology, University of Oslo, The National Hospital, N-0027, Oslo, Norway.

The increased density of jejunal intraepithelial lymphocytes (IEL) in coeliac disease (CD) is interesting in view of the possible T-cell involvement in the pathogenesis. In human peripheral lymphoid tissues and blood, about 95% of T-cells express the α/β T-cell receptor (TCRα/β). A second TCR termed τ/δ has been identified on a minor fraction of peripheral T-cells which are mostly CD4-8- ("double negative"). Human IEL have recently been shown to be mostly of the TCRα/β+CD8+ phenotype with only a small fraction of the TCRτ/δ+ variety. We have studied the expression of the TCRτ/δ on CD3+ IEL <u>in situ</u> by two-colour immunofluorescence on jejunal tissue sections from 24 patients with CD and 17 controls. The proportion of intraepithelial TCRτ/δ+ cells was significantly increased ($p<0.002$) in untreated (median 20%, range 11-53%) and treated CD (median 23%, range 16-55%) compared with controls (median 2%, range 0-39%). This subset was preferentially located within the epithelium rather than in the lamina propria. Paired staining showed that most (~90%) intraepithelial TCRτ/δ+ lymphocytes were CD8- in CD, and a remarkably large fraction (medain 67%, range 58-94%) expressed the Vδ1/Jδ1 or Vδ1/Jδ2-encoded epitope (MoAb δTCS1+). The intraepithelial TCRτ/δ+CD8-T-cell subset thus shows a particular association with CD.

INTRODUCTION

T cells recognize antigen by their TCR. In human peripheral lymphoid tissues and blood, about 95% of the T cells express a 90-kDa disulphide-linked heterodimer composed of α and ß chains. Most such TCRα/ß+ cells are either CD4+ or CD8+ and generally recognize antigenic peptides in the context of "self" major histocompatibility complex (MHC) class II or class I molecules, respectively. The second TCR termed τ/δ is expressed on a minor fraction (5%) of peripheral T cells (4). TCRτ/δ+ cells often lack CD4 and CD8 molecules and their antigenic repertoire and putative restriction elements are still obscure (1). Murine small intestinal epithelium has been claimed to contain exclusively a unique population of TCRτ/δ+CD8+ lymphocytes (2,6), whereas most human IEL are TCRα/ß+ with only a small fraction (<8%) TCRτ/δ+ cells (3, 5,7). To further characterize IEL and lamina propria T cells in CD, we used a two- colour immunofluorescence <u>in situ</u> method to examine the distribution of TCRτ/δ+ cells within the two tissue compartments.

MATERIALS AND METHODS

Tissue specimens

Biopsy specimens from the proximal small intestine were obtained from 5 chil-

M. L. Mearin and C. J. J. Mulder (eds.), Coeliac Disease, 71–75.

dren and 19 adult patients with CD, 13 untreated and 11 on a gluten-free diet. Histologically normal mucosa from 17 controls were included. Tissue specimens were oriented on a slice of carrot, embedded in OCT, snap-frozen in isopenthane that was cooled in liquid nitrogen, and stored at -70°C until cryo-sectioning as detailed elsewere (8). Jejunal biopsy specimens from nine of the patients were directly fixed in cold 96% ethanol for 18 h, dehydrated in absolute ethanol, cleared in xylene, embedded in paraffin for 3-4 hrs at 56°C, and stored at 4°C until sectioning.

Immunofluorescence staining

The details of the staining technique has been published elsewere (8). Briefly, 4 μm cryo-sections were incubated (1 h) with the combinations of unlabelled monoclonal antibody (MoAb) reagents listed in Table 1. MoAb TCRδ1 was combined with RIV9; MoAb TCRδ1 with BMA-081; MoAb ßF1 with RIV9. Secondary reagents were mixtures of either biotinylated (0.01 g/l) or FITC-conjungated (0.05 g/l) goat subclass-specific anti mouse IgG1, IgG2a or IgG3 (Southern Biotechnology, Birmingham, AL), followed by. Streptavidin-Texas Red (0.01 g/l; BRL, Gaithersburg, MD). MoAb anti-Leu-4 were used in combination with MoAb TCRδ1 on ethanol-fixed, paraffinembedded tissue in a sequential staining technique detailed previously (8). Similar methods were used to examine the percentage of TCRτ/δ+ cells that expressed the epitope for MoAb δTCS1.

Microscopy and cell enumeration

Immunofluorescence was examined at 480 times magnification in a Leitz Orthoplan microscope equipped with a Ploem-type vertical illuminator for selective observation of red, green, or blue emission. The count of CD3+TCRτ/δ+ IEL in cryo-sections and ethanol-fixed specimens were done by evaluating every CD3+ cell for TCRτ/δ expression.

TABLE I MOUSE MoAb USED IN THIS STUDY

MoAb	Speci-ficity	Sub-class	Dilu-tions	Source
TCRδ1	TCRτ/δ	IgG1	1:20	T Cell Sciences, Cambridge, MA
ßF1	TCRα/ß	IgG1	1:20	T Cell Sciences
δTCS1	Vδ1	IgG1	1:20	T Cell Sciences
Leu-4	CD3	IgG1	1:20	Becton Dickinson, Mountain View, CA
RIV9	CD3	IgG3	1:10	Sanbio, Am Uden, The Netherlands
BMA-081	CD8	IgG2a	1:40	Behring, Marburg, FRG

RESULTS

The percentage TCRτ/δ+ T cells and their CD8 expression

In each section every intraepithelial CD3+ cell (median 245; range, 59-642) and a random selection of CD3+ lamina propria lymphocytes (median, 154; range, 97-

378), were examined by the combination of MoAb to the constant TCRδ chain and to CD3. TCRγ/δ cells were mainly observed within the epithelium; only 2% (range, 0-10%) of the lamina propria CD3+ cells expressed TCRγ/δ.

FIGURE I

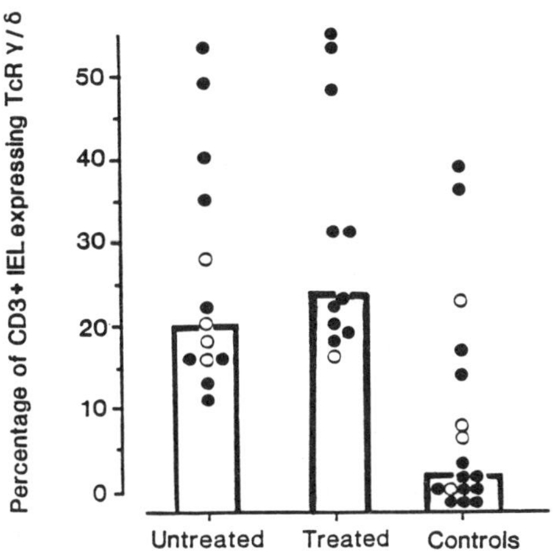

Scatter diagram of TCRγ/δ+ IEL distribution in children (o) and adults (●) with untreated (n=13) or treated (n=11) CD and controls with normal jejunal mucosa (n=17). Columns indicate medians.

TCRγ/δ+ IEL (median, 32; range 1-123) in CD and control specimens (13 of each category) were further examined for CD8 expression. Most TCRγ/δ+ IEL were CD8- both in CD (median 90%, range, 78-100%) and in the controls (median 75%, range, 34-100%). Too few TCRγ/δ+ cells (median 5%, range 0-26%) were observed in the lamina propria for conclusive evaluation of CD8 co-expression, but most of them were CD8 negative (median 94%, range 50-100%). A significant ($p<0.002$, Willcoxon two-tailed test) increase in the percentage TCRγ/δ+ IEL was observed in CD compared with controls, regardless of whether the patients were treated or not (Fig. 1). However, also a few controls had a high proportion of TCRγ/δ+ IEL.

The MoAb δTCS1+ T cell subset

In each tissue section every TCRγ/δ+ T cell was examined by sequential two-colour staining for reactivity with MoAb δTCS1, which was taken to indicate co-expression of the variable Vδ1/Jδ1 or Vδ1/Jδ2 gene products (11). This examination was performed on 13 specimens from CD and 5 controls. Most such IEL (median 67%, range 58%-90%) were MoAb δTCS1+, both in coeliac patients and controls. Approximately the same percentage of lamina propria TCRγ/δ+ cells were MoAb δTCS1+ (median 66%, range 42-88%).

DISCUSSION

An anatomical dichotomy in the distribution of T cells expressing TCRα/ß and TCRτ/δ has been proposed (10), based on reports showing that murine intestinal epithelium contained virtually only the latter subset (2,6). This concept has recently been shown not to hold true in man (3,5,7), as also confirmed in this study. However, the few TCRτ/δ+ IEL observed in controls were preferentially located within the epithelium. In addition, an increased percentage of TCRτ/δ+ IEL was observed in treated as well as in untreated coeliac patients. Similar results were recently reported by Spencer (18). This might reflect that TCRτ/δ+ cells are of particular importance in the pathogenesis of CD.

Between 30% and 90% of the TCRτ/δ+ cells in human peripheral blood have been reported to be CD4-8- (7). Intraepithelial TCRτ/δ+ cells were in this study generally found to be CD8 negative, both in controls (72%) and in CD (90%). This observation contrasts with the 100% CD8 expression reported for murine TCRτ/δ+ IEL (2,6), but it agrees with the reported increase of CD3+4-8- IEL in untreated and treated patients with CD (10,17).

About 70% of the TCRτ/δ+ cells both in the lamina propria and epithelium were found be MoAb δTCS1+. Less than 30% of TCRτ/δ cells in peripheral blood have been reported to express this epitope (7,12). Our finding may therefore reflect local clonal expansion of a particular subset of TCRτ/δ+ cells, but a similar high frequency of this phenotype has been reported in the thymus (12). TCRτ/δ+ lymphocytes comprise a separate sublinage of T cells with a mostly unknown antigenic repertoire and restriction elements (1). Intestinal TCRτ/δ+ IEL may primarily be directed against microorganisms, or perhaps be specialized for elimination of transformed, infected or otherwise "stressed" cells (9,13). Many TCRτ/δ+CD4-8- cell clones have been isolated and shown to exhibit both antigen-specific MHC-restricted as well as antigen-unspecific and MHC-unrestricted cytotoxicity against a variety of tumor cell lines (15).

Whether human TCRτ/δ+ IEL in CD are cytolytic remains to be shown. Perhaps they react with gluten peptides, which may be presented to them by the epithelial cells in the context of MHC or MHC-like molecules. When intestinal T cells are activated, lymphokine(s) may be released that cause the crypt epithelium to proliferate (14).

CD is strongly associated with a HLA-DQw2 heterodimer whether it is encoded in cis or trans (16). Subjects with certain MHC alleles in combination with an increased fraction of TCRτ/δ+ IEL may, therefore, be particularly susceptible to CD.

REFERENCES

1 Bluestone JA, Matis LA. TCRτ/δ-cells minor redundant T cell subset or specialized immune system component? J Immunol 1989;142:1785.

2 Bonneville M, Janeway CA, Ito K, Haser W, Ishida I, Nakanishi N, Tonegawa S. Intestinal intraepithelial lymphocytes are a distinct set of τδ T cells. Nature (London) 1988;336:479.

3 Brandtzaeg P, Halstensen TS, Scott H, Sollid LM, Valnes KN, Bosnes V. Epithelial homing of τ/δ T cells? Nature 1989;341:113.

4 Brenner MB, McLean J, Dialynas DP, Strominger JL, Smith JA, Owen FL, Seidman JG, Stephen IP, Rosen F, Krangel MS. Identification of a putative second T-cell receptor. Nature (London)

1986;322:145.

5 Bucy RP, Chen C-LH, Cooper MD. Tissue localization and CD8 accessory molecule expression of T$\tau\delta$ cells in humans. J Immunol 1989;142:3045.

6 Goodman T, Lefrancois L. Expression of the τ-δ T-cell receptor on intestinal CD8+ intra-epithelial lymphocytes. Nature (London) 1988;333:855.

7 Groh V, Porcelli S, Fabbi M, Lanier LL, Picker LJ, Anderson T, Warnke RA, Bhan AK, Strominger JL, Brenner MB. Human lymphocytes bearing T cell receptor τ/δ are phenotypically diverse and evenly distributed throughout the lymphoid system. J Exp Med 1989;169.

8 Halstensen TS, Scot H, Brandtzaeg P. Intraepithelial T Cells of the TcRτ/δ+CD8-and Vδ1/Jδ1+ Phenotypes are Increased in Coeliac Disease. Scand J Immunol 1989;30:665.

9 Janeway CA, Jones B, Hayday A. Specificity and function of T cells bearing $\tau\delta$ receptors. Immunol Today 1988;9:73.

10 Jenkins D, Goodall A, Scott BB. T-lymphocyte populations in normal and coeliac small intestinal mucosa defined by monoclonal antibodies. Gut 1986;27:1330.

11 Koning F, Knot M, Wassenaar F, Van den Elsen P. Phenotypical heterogeneity among human cell receptor τ/δ-expressing clones derived from peripherial blood. Eur J Immunol 1989:19,2099

12 Lanier LL, Ruitenberg JJ, Bolhuis RLH, Borst J, Phillips J, Testi R. Structural and serological heterogeneity of τ/δ T cells antigen receptor expression in thymus and peripherial Blood. Eur J Immunol 1988;18:985.

13 Lefrancois L, Goodman T. In vivo modulation of cytolytic activity and thy-1 expression in TCR-τ/δ+ intraepithelial lymphocytes. Science 1989;243:1716.

14 MacDonald TT, Spencer J. Evidence that activated mucosal T cells play a role in the pathogenesis of enteropathy in human small intestine. J Exp Med 1988;167:1341.

15 Raulet DH. Antigens for τ/δ T cells. Nature (London) 1989;339:42.

16 Sollid LM, Markussen G, Ek J, Gjerde H, Vardal F, Thorsby E. Evidence for a primary association of celiac disease to a particular HLA-DQ α/ß heterodimer. J Exp Med 1989;169:345.

17 Spencer J, MacDonald TT, Diss TO, Walker-Smith JA, Ciclitira PJ, Isaacson PG. Changes in intraepithelial lymphocyte subpopulations in coeliac disease and enteropathy associated T cell lymphoma (malignant histiocytosis of the intestine). Gut 1989;30:339.

18 Spencer J, Isaacson PG, Diss TO, MacDonald, TT. Expression of disulfide-linked and non-disulfide linked form of the T cell receptor τ/δ heterodimer in human intestinal intraepithelial lymphocytes Eur J Immunol 1989;19:1335.

INTESTINAL GAMMA/DELTA RECEPTOR BEARING T LYMPHOCYTES ARE INCREASED IN COELIAC DISEASE AND DERMATITIS HERPETIFORMIS.

E. Savilahti, A. Arato, T. Reunala, M. Verkasalo. Children's Hospital, University of Helsinki, Department of Dermatology, University of Tampere, Finland.

We studied the numbers of T cell receptor (TCR) gamma/delta (γ/δ) bearing lymphocytes in 45 jejunal specimens from 19 patients with coeliac disease (CD), 6 patients with dermatitis herpetiformis (DH), and 13 controls with normal jejunum and one patient with villous atrophy and severe food allergy. Monoclonal antibodies and a three-layer peroxidase staining method were used. In the lamina propria and epithelium of a normal jejunum and in the specimen of the patient with food allergy only low numbers of $\gamma/\delta+$ cells were seen. In the lamina propria of coeliac patients, the mean number of $\gamma/\delta+$ cells was significantly higher than in the controls before treatment, during gluten free diet and after the gluten challenge. Patients with DH were on normal diet; they showed a similar increase of $\gamma/\delta+$ cells as CD patients. In the jejunal surface and crypt epithelium of CD patients, the number of $\gamma/\delta+$ cells was elevated before and during gluten elimination and after the challenge test. In the epithelium, the absolute number of these cells remained constant during gluten elimination and provocation. In the specimens of DH patients a similar increase was seen; in both groups the mean number of $\gamma/\delta+$ was about 30% of that of CD3+ cells. We infer that the elevated population of $\gamma/\delta+$ T cells in the epithelium of CD and DH patients may play an important role in the pathogenesis of jejunal damage.

INTRODUCTION

The recently recognized T cell type bearing TCR γ/δ as a part of the CD3 complex (1,2) has not been assigned a specific role in the lymphoid tissue of man. In mice, TCR γ/δ cells have been found in abundance among the dendritic epidermal cells (3,4) and analysis of the surface receptor proteins of the intestinal intraepithelial T cells suggested that the majority of them could bear γ/δ receptors (5). In the normal human jejunum, the number of TCR γ/δ bearing cells seems to be low, both in the lamina propria and intraepithelially, according to recent studies (6-9). In jejunal mucosa TCR γ/δ cells form only as small percentage of the total number of CD3+ T cells as has been described for the peripheral blood and thymic lymphocytes, (6,10). In patients with CD, there is a significant increase in the absolute and proportionate counts of γ/δ TCR-bearing cells in the epithelium (7,11,12) and, according to our previous study (12), also in the lamina propria of the jejunum. The close relationship of CD and dermatitis herpetiformis (DH) (13,14) prompted us to study the numbers of γ/δ TCR bearing cells in the jejunum of patients with DH. We found an even more pronounced increase of TCR γ/δ bearing cells in the jejunum of DH patients than in coeliacs. Long lasting adherence to gluten free diet (GFD) had no influence on the density of TCR γ/δ cells.

M. L. Mearin and C. J. J. Mulder (eds.), Coeliac Disease, 77–84.

PATIENTS

Jejunal biopsy specimens of 22 patients with DH were avialable for the study. The diagnosis of DH was based on the finding of typical skin lesions and the demonstration of granular IgA deposits in the immunofluorescent study of the unaffected skin biopsy (13,15). Of the specimens, 13 were taken before any dietary treatment at the mean age of 40 years, and 9 during a gluten free diet at the mean age of 39 years. Patients had been on the gluten free diet for a period from 1 to 15 years. Findings were compared with those in 25 jejunal specimens from 19 paediatric patients with CD (12); 9 were taken before treatment at a mean age of 5.3 years, 8 were taken during gluten-free diet (mean age 12.1 years), and 8 after a gluten challenge resulting in villous atrophy (mean age 12.2 years). As controls we studied 13 histologically normal jejunal specimens taken from children at a mean age of 8.2 years as a part of the evaluation of their asymptomatic growth failure (16).

METHODS

Evaluation of biopsies: the jejunal biopsy specimens were divided and a part was processed for routine histology. The heights of the villi and the depths of the crypts were measured (15), and when the ratio of villus height to crypt depth was <2, the specimens were graded as showing subtotal villous atrophy (SVA), ratio 2.0-3.0 as partial villous atrophy (PVA) and ratio >3 as normal (N). Tissue processing: another part of the biopsy specimen was freshly embedded in OCT compound and stored at -70 C. Five μ cryostat serial sections were fixed in acetone for 10 minutes, then in chloroform for 30 minutes, and washed three times in Tris buffer pH 7.4. Immunohistochemical staining: after removing the buffer sections were covered with the diluted monoclonal antibodies in Tris-buffer for 16 hours. Endogenous peroxidase was blocked by incubation in 0.5% peroxide for 30 minutes. To stain monoclonal antibodies, a Vectastain Elite ABC kit (PK-6102, Vectro Laboratories, Burlinghame, CA.) was used according to the instructions of the manufacturer. Positively stained cells were counted with a light microscope through a calibrated graticule using 900x magnification (16,17). Monoclonal antibodies: monoclonal antibody TCRδ1 (T cell Sciences Inc. Cambridge, MA), recognizing constant region of δ-chain of TCR (18,19) and all τ/δ cells (6,20), and antibody βF1, reacting virtually with all α/β TCR molecules (20) were used in dilution 1:100. Monoclonal antibody Leu4 (anti-CD3, Beckton-Dickinson, Mountain View, Ca) was used in dilution 1:400. Statistical analysis: the number of cells in the study specimens were compared with those of the controls using Student's t-test.

RESULTS

TCR τ/δ bearing lymphocytes in the lamina propria of jejunum: patients with DH had more τ/δ cells in the lamina propria than the controls, and the increase was similar to that observed in the coeliacs (Table 1). The numbers were influenced neither by the diet the patients were on, nor by the morphology of the biopsy specimens (data not shown).

TABLE I τ/δ, α/β AND CD3 POSITIVE CELLS/MM2 OF THE LAMINA PROPRIA OF JEJUNUM.

Group	Number	τ/δ	α/β	CD3
Controls	13	69	1613	1473
DH patients on				
- normal diet	13	139*	1423	1778
- GFD	9	141	1582	2022
Coeliacs on				
- normal diet	25	198#	1303	1340
- on GFD	8	212*	1220	1354

* = -$p<0.05$; # = -$p<0.0001$ as compared with controls; DH = Dermatitis herpetiformis; GFD = Gluten-free diet.

TCR τ/δ bearing lymphocytes in the jejunal epithelium: in the surface epithelium of specimens taken during gluten containing diet, in patients with DH, the density of τ/δ cells was greater than in the controls ($p<0.0001$) and in the coeliacs ($p<0.005$) (Figure I). The τ/δ cells formed on average 40% of the CD3+ cells, and their density was similar in all morphological groups (9 subtotal villous atrophy, 2 partial villous atrophy and 2 normal). The density of α/β intraepithelial lymphocytes was also highest in DH patients with subtotal villous atrophy ($p<0.0001$ compared to controls, and $p<0.05$ compared to coeliac patients with villous atrophy).
During GFD, the density of τ/δ cells was also highest in the specimens of DH patients (Figure II), ($p<0.05$ when comparing the specimens with normal villous structure of DH patients with those of coeliacs). In the specimens of DH patients on GFD the mean percentage of τ/δ cells of the CD3 cells was 48%. The numbers of α/β+ cells did not differ signficantly between the patient groups.

FIGURE I

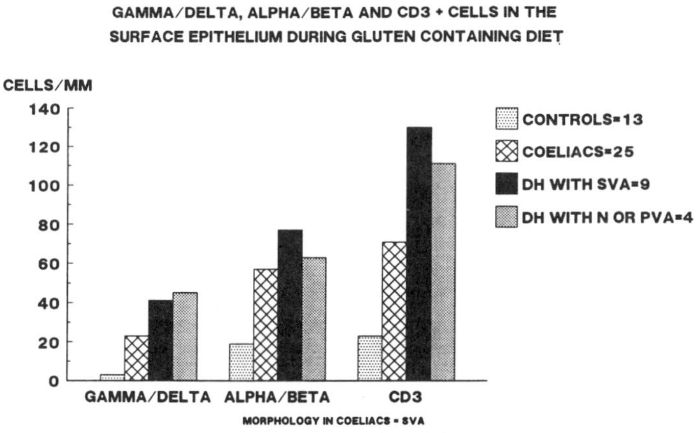

FIGURE II

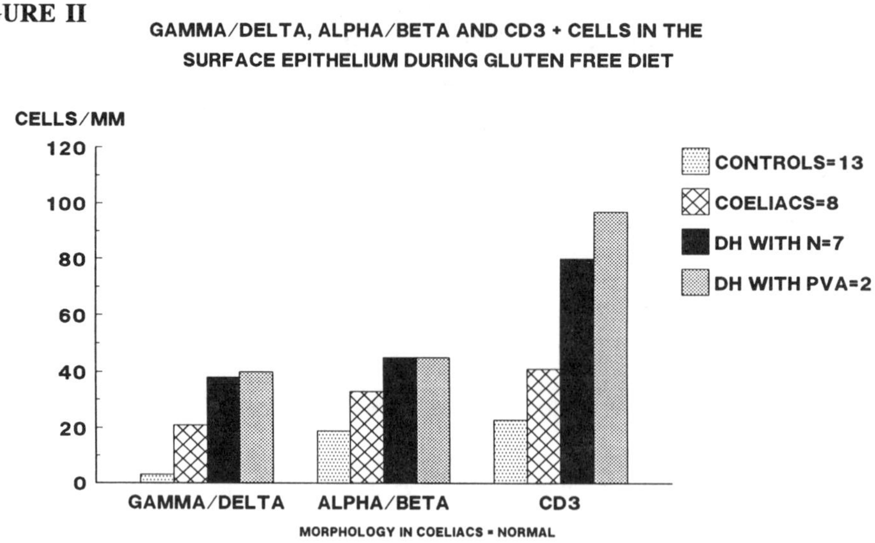

FIGURE III

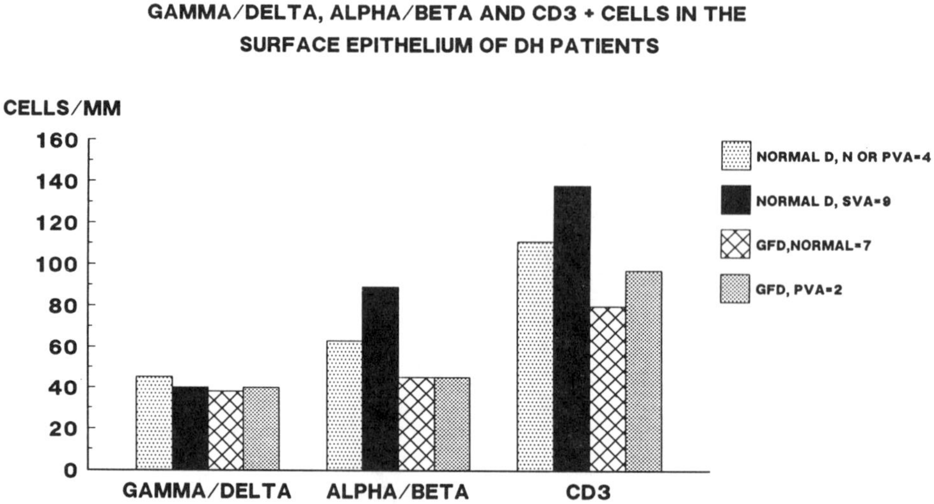

The densities of τ/δ cells in the jejunal epithelium remain high in DH patients regardless of dietary treatment or the severity of the jejunal damage (Figure III). The numbers of α/β cells are significantly lower in morphologically normal specimens taken from DH patients during GFD than in specimens with total villous atrophy taken during normal diet ($p<0.001$). In the morphologically normal specimens of DH patients the mean density of τ/δ cells (38/mm) was close to that of α/β cells (45/mm).

Age and the density of TCR τ/δ bearing lymphocytes: we studied the possible association of age with the density of τ/δ cells in the epithelium, because the ages of DH patients were higher (mean age 40 years) than those of the paediatric group of coeliac patients (mean age 10 years). In the specimens of coeliacs no significant association with age was seen (Figure IV, R=0.34, p>0.05). The densities in specimens of older DH patients seemed to be lower than in the younger ones, but the association was not significant (Figure V, R=-0.33, p>0.05).

FIGURE IV

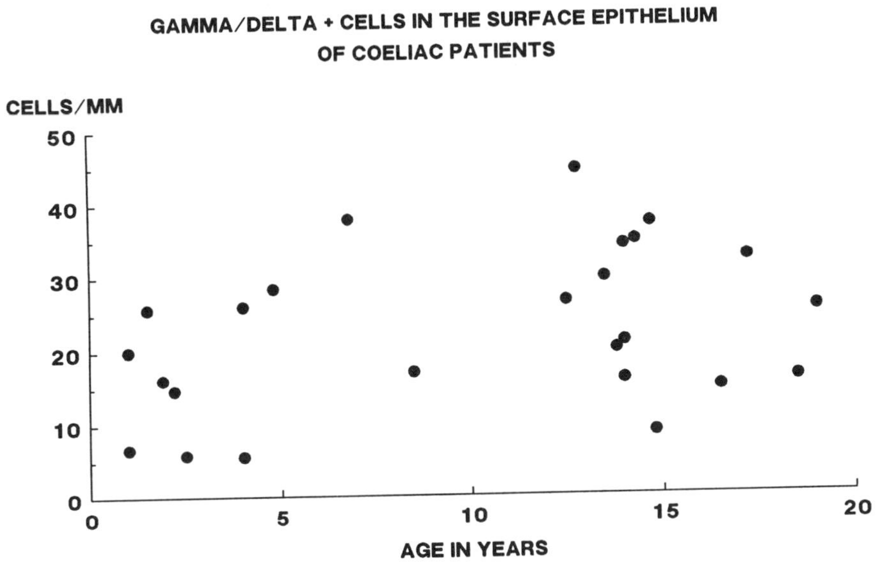

FIGURE V

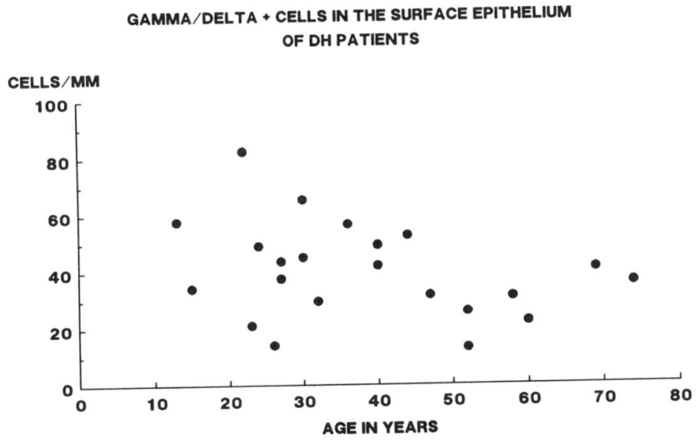

DISCUSSION

Our main finding is a significant increase of τ/δ cells in the jejunum of patients with DH. In the lamina propria the increase was of the same order as in coeliacs, but in the epithelium patients with DH had more τ/δ cells than coeliacs, both during normal gluten containing diet and GFD. In DH patients the density was quite similar in the epithelium irrespective of the diet or the morphology of the jejunum. The relative density of τ/δ cells was highest during GFD; they were nearly as frequent as α/β cells.

It has been speculated that τ/δ cells may have a special function in the defence of mucosal surfaces by eliminating infected or otherwise damaged epithelial cells (21). TCR τ/δ bearing cells can exert cytolytic activity against tumor cells, which is not restricted by MHC class I and II molecules (22,23), and also towards IgG Fc receptor-bearing target cells (24) when first activated with monoclonal antibody to CD3. Clearly, both types of cytolytic reaction could play a role in the pathogenesis of the jejunal damage seen always in CD and in the majority of patients with DH (13,15,25). It may be speculated that if τ/δ cells are stimulated by fractions of gluten or intraluminal microbial antigens, they may become cytotoxic to the altered surface epithelial cells. DH and CD are associated with the same MHC antigens (13,26-28). These, or other related restricting surface antigens may show high affinity to digested fractions of gluten and, together with specific antibodies, render them targets for cytolysis.

Our present results, on the other hand suggest that τ/δ cells are not involved in the elimination of epithelial cells, which probably produces the jejunal damage typical of CD and DH. The numbers of τ/δ cells were similar with maintained intestinal structure during gluten containing diet and those with severe villous atrophy. As in CD (12), the gluten elimination in DH did not change their density, while the numbers of α/β cells changed conform to dietary treatment both in DH (present study) and in CD (12).

Furthermore, in other diseases with villous atrophy, such as tropical sprue (7) and severe intestinal food allergy (12), the number of τ/δ cells has been found to be normal. The presence of increased numbers of τ/δ TCR positive cells could be due to the immune abnormality common to CD and DH and expressed as similar HLA-D associations (13,26-28). Whether the greater density of τ/δ cells of DH patients has any role in the accumulation of immunocomplexes in their skin, or in the better maintenance of intestinal integrity of DH patients, can only be speculated.

REFERENCES

1 Bank I, Depinho RA, Brenner MB et al. A functional T3 molecule associated with a novel heterodimer on the surface of immature human thymocytes. Nature 1986;322:179-181.

2 Brenner MB, McLean J, Dialynas DP et al. Identification of a putative second T-cell receptor. Nature 1986;322:145-149.

3 Konig F, Stingl G, Yokoyama WM et al. Identification of T3-associated gammadelta T cell receptor in Thy-1+ dendritic epidermal cell lines. Science 1987;236:834-836.

4 Kuziel WA, Takashima A, Bonyhadi M et al. Regulation of T-cell receptor gamma-chain RNA expression in murine Thy-1+ dendritic epidermal cells. Nature 1987;328:263-266.

5 Goodman T, Lefrancois L. Expression of the gamma/delta T-cell receptor on intestinal CD8+

intraepithelial lymphocytes. Nature 1988;333:855-857.
6 Groh V, Porcell S, Fabbi M et al. Human lymphocytes bearing T cell receptor gamma/delta are phenotypically diverse and evenly distributed throughout the lymphoid system. Journal of Experimental Medicine 1989;169:1277-1294.
7 Spencer J, Isaacson PG, Dis TC, MacDonald TT. Expression of disulfide-linked and non-disulfide-linked forms of the T cell receptor gamma/delta heterodimer in human intestinal intraepithelial lymphocytes. European Journal of Immunology 1989;19:1335-1338.
8 Brandtzaeg P, Bosnes V, Halstensen TS et al. T lymphocytes in human gut epithelium preferentially express the alpha/beta antigen receptor and are often CD45/UCHL1-positive. Scandinavian Journal of Immunology 1989;30:123-128.
9 Bucy RP, Chen C-LH, Cooper MD. Tissue localization and CD8 accessory molecule expression of T-gamma/delta cells in humans. Journal of Immunology 1989;141:3045-3049.
10 Brenner MB, Strominger JL, Krangel MS. The gamma/delta receptor. Advances in Immunology 1988;43:133-192.
11 Halstensen TS, Scott H, Brandtzaeg T. Intraepithelial T cells of TcRgamma/ delta+CD8- and Vdelta1/Jdelta1+ phenotypes are increased in coeliac disease. Scandinavian Journal of Immunology 1989;30:665-672.
12 Savilahti E, Arato A, Verkasalo M. Intestinal gamma/delta receptor bearing T lymphocytes in coeliac disease and inflammatory bowel disease in children. Constant increase in coeliac disease. Submitted to Pediatric Research: in press.
13 Hall RP. The pathogenesis of dermatitis herpetoformis: recent advances. Journal of the American Academy of Dermatology 1987;16:1129-1144.
14 Savilahti E, Reunala T. Is dermatitis herpetiformis a gluten sensitive enteropathy? International Journal of Dermatology: in press.
15 Reunala T. Gluten-free diet in dermatitis herpetiformis. II. Morphological and immunological findings in the skin and small intestine of 12 patients and matched controls. British Journal of Dermatology 1978;98:69-78.
16 Verkasalo M, Arato A, Savilahti E, Tainio V-M. Effect of diet and age on jejunal and circulating lymphocyte subsets in children with coeliac disease. Gut 1990;31:422-425.
17 Arato A, Savilahti E, Tainio V, Klemola T. Immunohistochemical study of lymphoplasmacytic infiltrate and epithelial HLA-DR expression in the rectal and colonic mucosae of children with ulcerative colitis. Journal of Pediatric Gastroentrology and Nutrition 1989;8:172-180.
18 Band H, Hochstenbach F, McLean J, Hata S, Krangel MS, Brenner MB. Immunochemical proof that a novel rearranging gene encodes the T cell receptor delta subunit. Science 1987;238:682-4.
19 Tribel F, Hercend T. Subpopulations of human peripheral T gamma delta lymphocytes. Immunology Today 1989;10:186-188.
20 Faure F, Jitsukawa S, Triebel F, Hercend T. Characterization of human peripheral lymphocytes expressing the CD3-gamma/delta complex with anti-receptor monoclonal antibodies. Journal of Immunology 1988;141:3357-3360.
21 Janeway CAJ, Jones B, Hayday A. Specificity and function of T cells bearing gammadelta receptors. Immunology Today 1989;9:73-6.
22 Borst J, van de Griend RJ, van Oostveen JW et al. A T-cell receptor gamma/CD3 complex found on cloned functional lymphocytes. Nature 1987;325:683-688.
23 Ciccione E, Ferrini S, Bottino C et al. Monoclonal antibody specific for a common determinant of the human T cell receptor gamma/delta directly activate CD3+ WT31- lymphocytes to express their functional program(s). Journal of Experimental Medicine 1988;168:1-11.
24 van de Griend RJ, Tax WJM, van Krimpen BA et al. Lysis of tumor cells by CD3+8-16+ T cell receptor alphabeta-clones, regulated via CD3 and CD16 activation sites, recombinant interleukin 2, and interferon beta. Journal of Immunology 1987;138:1627-1633.
25 Reunala T, Kosnai I, Karpati S et al. Dermatitis herpetiformis: jejunal findings and skin response to gluten free diet. Archives of Diseases in Childhood 1984;59:517-522.
26 Mearin ML, Biemond I, Peña AS et al. HLA-DR phenotypes in Spanish coeliac children: their contribution to the understanding of the genetics of the disease. Gut 1983;24:532-538.
27 Sollid LM, Markussen G, Ek J et al. Evidence for a primary association of coeliac disease to

a particular HLA-DQ alpha/beta heterodimer. Journal of Experimental Medicine 1989;169:345-350.

28 Hall R, Sanders ME, Duquesnoy RJ et al. Alterations in HLA-DP and HLA-DQ antigen frequency in patients with dermatitis herpetiformis. Journal of Investigative Dermatology 1989;93:501-505.

DETECTING GLUTEN AND RELATED PROLAMINS IN FOOD.

John H Skerritt and Amanda S Hill, CSIRO Wheat Research Unit, Division of Plant Industry, PO Box 7, North Ryde, NSW 2113, Australia.

The universal approach to the management of coeliac disease is the exclusion of gluten from wheat, rye and barley from the diet. However, adherence to "gluten-free" diets is difficult because:
1. Labelling legislation in many countries allows incomplete description of food components. 2. Gluten can be found in unexpected sources, for example, as a binder in pharmaceuticals, confectionery, desserts, flavourings and sauces or as a protein extender in meat products. 3. In many cases the composition of raw materials is not exactly known to food manufacturers. 4. Current gluten content rules are imprecise.
Existing techniques such as polyacrylamide gel electrophoresis, HPLC and microscopy are not quantitative, are slow or expensive and are often quite unreliable with cooked or processed foods. Conventional (polyclonal) antibody tests can only provide accurate results with uncooked products such as "gluten-free" bakery mixes. These antibodies can be hard to standardize or produce in large quantities. Two simple monoclonal antibody-based test kits have been developed for the detection of gluten in foods. The "Gluten Lab-Test" is the first method developed which is able to quantify gluten in all types of uncooked, cooked and processed foods and is intended for use by food manufacturers and government laboratories. The second, "Rapid Gluten Test Kit" provides rapid, qualitative or semi-quantitative results and is suitable for home use by coeliacs, clinic use by dietitians, or in-process quality control. We have selected antibodies to certain heat-stable omega-gliadins. The advantage of these antibodies is that they bind to those proteins that are not denatured by heating during baking, processing or cooking of foods. The monoclonal antibodies used in these tests were selected such that they bound to certain prolamins from bread wheat, durum wheat, triticale, rye and barley but not to proteins from maize or rice. The antibodies do not bind to oats which lack heat-stable omega-prolamins. Oats are usually easily identified in foods and, indeed, are consumed by many coeliacs. Both tests are based on a two-site method of enzyme-immunoassay. Using the laboratory test, food samples are extracted in 40% ethanol, centrifuged and diluted in buffer. The diluted food extract is incubated with the immobilized antibody. After washing, a horseradish peroxidase-labelled antibody is added, followed by substrate. The maximun sensitivity of the assay is 0.001% gluten. The rapid test is the first food test of its type which will allow individuals to monitor their diets. With this test, foods are coarsely ground, and gluten extracted by shaking for 60 seconds in the extractant provided, and a drop of sample is added to the detection tube and mixed 90 seconds. The antibody solution is added, the tube mixed, a test stick washed under tap water, and transferred to a second tube.
Presence of gluten in the food results in the development of a blue colour. A preformed coloured standard corresponding to results obtained with "just acceptable" amounts of gluten is provided in the kit for comparison. Prototypes of the rapid test kit were successfully trailled by over 50 Australian participants in 1989. It is hoped

M. L. Mearin and C. J. J. Mulder (eds.), Coeliac Disease, 85–94.

that the availability of both tests will not only make the quality of gluten-free food more reliable, but improve the dietary management of coeliac disease.

INTRODUCTION

Although it is now forty years since Dicke and others identified gluten proteins as being the causative agents of coeliac disease (CD), the primary means of treatment of the condition remains the enforcement of a strict gluten-free diet. This is because our understanding of the molecular mechanisms of action of gluten polypeptides upon the coeliac intestinal mucosa remain very incomplete, so "cure" of CD by immunotherapy or pharmacological means is not currently possible. Clinical experience suggests that while bread wheat, durum wheat and rye are quite coeliac-toxic, barley is less so, while the toxicity of oats is somewhat controversial (1,2). Maize and rice (and probably millet and sorghum) are non-toxic. These differences in toxicities arise from an interplay of differences in the amino acid sequences and thus structures of the various prolamins in the different cereals, and the amounts of these prolamins. For example, oats may have slight toxicity because the proportion of prolamin in the grain is relatively low and the oat prolamins are only slightly similar to wheat prolamins; maize may be non-toxic even though it has the same amount of prolamin as wheat because the prolamins are structurally very different in the two species.

The presence of gluten in foods is usually hard to detect simply by eye or taste, and the adherence to "gluten-free" diets is therefore difficult because:

1. Labelling legislation in many countries allows incomplete description of food components.
2. Gluten can be found in unexpected sources, for example, as a binder in pharmaceuticals, confectionery, desserts, flavourings and sauces or as a protein extender in meat products.
3. In many cases the composition of raw materials is not exactly known to food manufacturers.
4. Current gluten content rules are imprecise. WHO/FAO Codex Alimentarius guidelines state that products containing greater than 0.3% protein from coeliac-toxic cereals cannot be labelled as being "gluten-free". However it is the actual gluten protein content, not the total cereal protein content, that of course determines coeliac-toxicity.

These considerations have led to considerable effort in developing methods for identification or quantification of gluten in foods, including special dietary foods claimed to be "gluten-free". Protein chemical techniques such as polyacrylamide gel electrophoresis, HPLC and microscopy are not quantitative, are slow or expensive and are often quite unreliable with cooked or processed foods. Long-established immunochemical methods based on antigen diffusion in gels perform best with water-soluble proteins, yet gluten and related cereal storage proteins are insoluble in aqueous buffers.

However, one of the first tests for gliadin in foods was the double diffusion method of Zareba (3); in this study, normal and gluten-free breads were extracted under alkaline conditions. Keyser and Mahler (4) also used alkaline conditions for similar work with starch preparations, although Lietze (5) was able to use neutral phosphate-buffer extracts for detection of gluten in special dietary breads. Guenther (6) analysed a large number of meat samples for soya and wheat protein by single radial immunodiffusion using commercially-available antisera. Baudner (7), Kaczkowski (8) and Bauer and Stachelberger (9) have described diffusion-in-gel methods (including immunoelectrophoresis) for qualitative or semi-quantitative estimation of gliadin in foods, including bakery products.

RADIO-IMMUNOASSAYS AND ENZYME-IMMUNOASSAYS FOR GLUTEN IN FOODS

In recent years, several groups have described very sensitive enzyme- or radio-immunoassays for gluten proteins. Like the diffusion-in-gel assays, competition and sandwich-enzyme immunoassays require some solubility of gliadin under "physiological" pH and salt concentrations, but because of the considerably greater sensitivity of the newer assays, this is usually readily achievable. Ciclitira and Lennox (10) described an assay using radio-labelled A-gliadin, with rabbit antisera and Staphylococcus Aureus to precipitate immune complexes. The antisera detected mainly alpha- and beta-gliadins, and qualitative detection of gliadin was possible after baking. This antiserum did not detect prolamins from other coeliac-toxic cereals. Analysis of some supposedly gluten-free products by this assay demonstrated that at least one product contained unacceptably high amounts (6.5mg/g) of gliadin (10).

Windemann and co-workers (11) described elegant heterogeneous enzyme- immunoassays suitable for quantifying either alpha-gliadin or whole gliadin. More recently, these workers applied their sandwich enzyme-immunoassay methods to the detection of gliadins in a range of unheated foods (12). The assay did not detect a range of non-gluten proteins, and recovery after extraction of uncooked foods with ethanol was good, except for those foods containing cocoa, coffee or tea. Their antiserum to alpha-gliadin was overly-specific, not cross-reacting even with rye. Another problem with such specific antisera was that differences in antibody binding to gliadins from different varieties of wheat was found.

More recently, other workers (13-15) have developed sandwich enzyme-immunoassays for gliadin, using either two polyclonal antibodies or one polyclonal and one monoclonal antibody. The polyclonal antibody test was very sensitive, detecting less than 0.5 ng of gliadin, however, since maize proteins were weakly detected, Troncone and co-workers (13) conceded that the method "cannot be indiscriminantly used to assess the suitability of gliadin-free foods for coeliac patients". The monoclonal antibodies used by Freedman (14) cross- reacted with rye, barley and oat prolamins, although the extent of reaction with rye was one-fiftieth that of wheat. As there is no clinical evidence to suggest that rye is significantly less toxic to coeliac patients than wheat (16), the test may only give useful results with uncooked, wheat-based products.

DETERMINATION OF GLUTEN IN COOKED OR PROCESSED FOODS

A major problem with each one of the enzyme-immunoassays described above, and with the earlier immunodiffusion assays is their unsuitability for use with cooked or processed foods. Although high-mobility (alpha- and beta-) gliadin components are likely the most toxic gliadins in CD (10,17) and their extractability and immunoreactivity is decreased upon heating (18,19), cooked foods containing gluten retain their toxicity. In contrast, milk whey proteins such as beta-lactoglobulin lose both their antigenicity and allergenicity following heat treatments (20).

Low mobility (omega-) gliadins are very heat-stable, most probably owing to their secondary structure and low contents of sulfur-containing amino acids and of heat-reactive amino acids such as lysine. We have described the isolation and characterisation of a number of omega-gliadin-binding monoclonal antibodies (21,22). Some of these antibodies also cross-react appropriately with prolamins from different cereals. Of several hundred monoclonal antibodies to wheat proteins, only a few were obtained with appropriate specificity, affinity, isotype and stability to conjugation and storage for use in robust commercial kits. The (patented) advantage of these antibodies is that they bind to those proteins that are not denatured by heating during baking, processing or cooking of foods. Unlike other methods, this enables accurate quantification of gluten in all types of foods. The monoclonal antibodies used in these tests were selected such that they bound to certain prolamins from bread wheat, durum wheat, triticale, rye and barley but not to proteins from maize or rice, and showed little difference in binding to different cultivars of wheat, barley and rye.

Initially, using the lower affinity antibodies, we developed simple qualitative or quantitative enzyme-immunoassays to detect gluten proteins adsorbed to nitrocellulose disks or strips following their soaking in food extracts (19,23,24). A direct antigen-adsorption assay of this type was possible since the gliadin-binding capacity of nitrocellulose disks is about 50-fold higher than that of plastic microwells (26). Other workers (26) have also described a dot-immunoassay using a monoclonal antibody to gliadin, but the specificity of this antibody for high-mobility gliadin will render this particular test being suitable only for uncooked, wheat-based foods. However, we did not advocate the routine use of these nitrocellulose disk tests for use in gluten determination assays. This is because the disks are somewhat difficult to manipulate in large numbers and high concentrations of monoclonal antibody were required.

Over the last three years, using higher-affinity omega-gliadin binding antibodies, we have now developed simple ELISA microwell- and tube-based assays for gluten determination. Two simple monoclonal antibody-based test kits have been developed for the detection of gluten in foods. The "Gluten Lab-Test" is the first method developed which is able to quantify gluten in all types of uncooked, cooked and processed foods. The second, "Rapid Gluten Test Kit" provides rapid, qualitative or semi-quantitative results and is suitable for home use or in-process quality control by food and wheat starch manufacturers.

Both tests are based on a two-site method of enzyme-immunoassay (Fig. I). Using the laboratory test, results are obtained in under 2 hours. Food samples are extracted in 40% ethanol, centrifuged and diluted in buffer. The diluted food extract is incubated with the microwell-immobilized antibody forming a gluten antigen-antibody complex. After washing steps, a horseradish peroxidase-labelled antibody is added which couples to the fixed gluten antigen. Further washing is carried out before substrate is added and incubated for 10 minutes. The product absorbance is proportional to the (log) gluten content of sample. The maximum sensitivity of the assay at 1/5 sample dilution is 0.002% gluten. Table I indicates just a few of a considerably larger range of foods that have been tested in the assay. Foods containing widely differing gluten contents can be assayed by simply changing the dilution factor. The test reliably detects gluten and gluten-like proteins from wheat, rye and barley in a wide range of raw or cooked foods, including specialty coeliac products, baked goods, processed meats, soups, confectionery and analgesics. The only interference seen in these tests from other food components was from polyphenol-containing ingredients such as cocoa or coffee. This interference has been removed by addition of of polyphenol-binding proteins to the food sample (11) or more simply by modification of the food extractant (Skerritt, Hill, unpublished). There is no complex work-up or preparation of samples, therefore allowing many samples to be tested simultaneously. The test kit has been designed so as not to require sophisticated equipment; all that is required are automatic pipettes, a spectrophotometer and a bench-top centrifuge.

FIGURE I METHOD FOR GLUTEN QUANTIFICATION IN FOODS

1. Food extracted in 40% Ethanol.
   Extract centrifuged and diluted in buffer

2. Incubation of diluted food extract
   with the monoclonal antibody (MCA)
   immobilized into the micro-well,
   forming gluten antigen-antibody complex.

3. Addition and incubation of labelled MCA.

4. Unbound food components removed by washing.
   Substrate added.

5. After stopping colour development,
   product absorbance is proportional
   to (log) gluten content of sample.

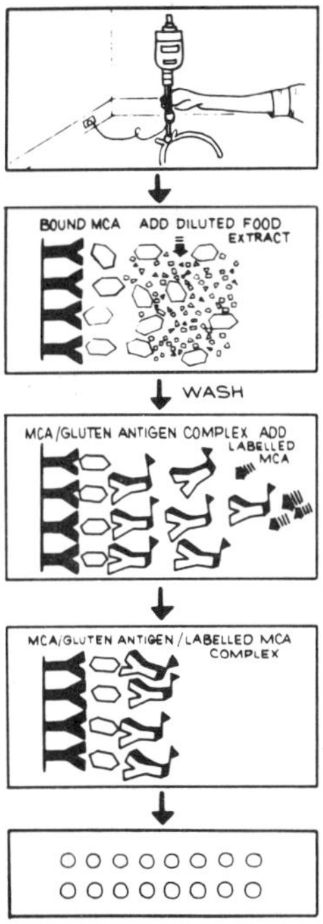

TABLE I GLUTEN CONTENT OF SELECTED FOODS MEASURED USING THE LABORATORY TEST

Food	Food Extract Dilution Tested	ELISA Absorbance	Gluten (%)
Maize starch (0.30% total protein)	50	0.03	n.d.
Wheat starches			
1 (0.24% total protein)	50	0.06	n.d.
2 (0.32% total protein)	50	0.34	0.03
3 (0.43% total protein)	50	0.78	0.12
Baking mixes labelled as "gluten-free"			
1	50	0.08	n.d.
2	50	1.05	0.30
3	50	0.33	0.03
Plain flour (cake type)	5000	0.63	7.2
Plain flour (bread type)	5000	0.81	12
Breakfast cereals labelled as "gluten-free"			
rice-based	50	0.03	n.d.
containing wheat germ	50	0.71	0.09
Baked foods			
bread crumbing mix	2500	0.85	7.3
sweet biscuit	2500	0.64	3.7
cracker	2500	0.62	3.5
crispbread	2500	0.33	1.5
Baby foods			
beef-based, no thickener	50	0.00	n.d.
chicken-based, thickener	50	1.10	0.40
Processed meats			
cooked beef product1	500	0.03	n.d.
2	500	0.73	1.0
3	2500	0.95	10
ham sausage	500	0.38	0.40
Soups - vegetable-based			
1	50	0.02	n.d.
2	50	1.08	0.39
Confectionery			
caramel1	50	0.05	n.d.
2	500	0.83	1.4
chocolate	500	0.22	0.20
Other food protein sources			
soy flour	50	0.00	n.d.
egg	50	0.00	n.d.
milk powder	50	0.00	n.d.

n.d. = not detectable (< 0.016%)

We have recently completed an international AOAC (Association of Official Analytical Chemists) collaborative trial of the kit and the method now has Official First Action approval. Fifteen participants in the USA and Europe completed analyses of five pre-trial samples (including wheat starches, processed meats and a flour sample), and thirteen trial samples (including wheat and maize starches, special dietary baking mixes, wheat flours, cookies, a soup and several cooked meat-gluten blends). All samples were analysed twice, and the sample set contained three pairs of "blind duplicate" samples. Gluten was either absent or present at between 0.02% and 11% by weight. Accuracy and precision results obtained were quite good. For accuracy, results obtained were 88-105% of actual, and for precision, the relative standard deviation of repeatability was 14-16% and the relative standard deviation of reproductibility was 24-56%. Lowest precision was obtained with analyses of small (1 gram) samples of meat products, in which gluten was shown to be unevenly distributed. In general, however, the precision results were quite acceptable for a method intended for analyses in a very wide range of food matrices, for a substance, present at concentrations varying over three orders of magnitude.

OTHER APPLICATIONS OF THE GLUTEN LABORATORY TEST

The laboratory kit has a number of other applications in the food, baking and cereal processing industries, including:

1. Measuring the total gluten content of flours or baked products (bread, bagels,pizza bases, pasta products), which has major effects on product texture, mouthfeel and keeping qualities. In raw materials, gluten content can be rapidly measured using the kit without need for gluten washing and Kjeldahl nitrogen analysis or alternatively performing calculations based on approximate protein content of non-flour components in baked goods. The test also enables gluten contents to be measured, for the first time, in finished products, allowing for new opportunities in product development and quality control.

2. Monitoring of starch quality with respect to gluten content. Other technologies can only measure total protein or nitrogen content of starches, while it is the gluten content that determines suitability of a starch for special dietary foods, baby foods or as a filler in pharmaceuticals. The gluten content of a starch also affects the degree of treatment required to remove nitrogenous material in glucose and dextrin production.

3. Monitoring the efficiency of gluten washing in starch/gluten manufacture. The kit can analyse effluent (monitoring gluten losses) and wet or dry glutens and starches.

4. The kit is suitable for use with both uncooked product mixes and baked or processed products such as processed meats. This can help the cereal manufacturer work together with meat processors, pet food manufacturers and other customers in developing optimised product formulations. Meat products

can be checked to ensure they fulfil meat- and non-meat protein content requirements.

5. Finally, the kit can be used by the manufacturer to monitor the gluten contents of types of foods where there is a market advantage in labelling them as being gluten-free, for example baby and infant foods, some health foods and pharmaceuticals.

Government laboratories can also use the kits for regulatory purposes since detection of gluten in foods is necessary:

1. To check the labelling of "gluten-free" special dietary foods.
2. For monitoring of illegal additions of cereals to meat products, or for in-house quality control of processed meats or confectionery for human or pet-food use. Many processed foods contain cereal proteins, to act in products as binders to improve texture, aid water and fat retention and, as extenders, lower the cost of the finished product. There are legal maximum levels of cereal and other non-meat proteins for incorporation in processed meats in almost all developed countries.

"HOME" OR "RAPID" TESTS FOR GLUTEN IN FOODS

The rapid test is designed for use in a home or office situation by gastroenterologists, dietitians and most importantly, by coeliacs themselves, and is the first food test of its type which will allow individuals to monitor their diets (Table II).
With this test, foods are coarsely ground, and gluten extracted by shaking for 60 seconds in the extractant provided, and a drop of sample and two drops of antibody are added to the coated tube and mixed for 3 minutes. The tube is then shaken, unbound components tipped out and the tube washed under tap water, and finally substrate is then added.

Presence of gluten in the food results in the development of a blue colour within seconds of addition of colour developer (enzyme substrate). A pre-formed coloured standard corresponding to results obtained with "just acceptable" amounts of gluten is provided in the kit for comparison. Prototypes of the rapid test kit were successfully trialled by over 50 Australian participants, including coeliacs, dietitians and food industry laboratories early in 1989.
There are two requirements of "home test" for gluten, additional to those for the laboratory test. In some cases, unopened home test kits must be stable for several months at room temperature for simplicity of storage, marketing and shipping, and the price per kit must be somewhat lower than that of the laboratory kit, since in most cases it will be members of the public, rather than companies or government laboratories that will be purchasing the home kit. This presents quite a challenge, as for example, the other antibody-based home kits that are commonly available to the public, namely home pregnancy test kits (which measure urinary human chorionic gonadotrophin) retail for between US$12 and $25 per test. Clearly such a price per

test for a home gluten test would not be sustainable, although it is expected that coeliacs and gluten-allergic individuals will perform a greater number of gluten tests per capita than pregnancy tests per annum.

TABLE II CRITICAL COMPARISON OF "LABORATORY" AND "HOME" ELISA TEST KITS FOR GLUTEN IN FOODS

	Laboratory test	Home test
Laboratory equipment needed?	Yes	No
Quantitative?	Yes	Semi-quantitative between 0.005-0.1% gluten
Time required?	2 hrs	5 mins
Suitable for simultaneous analysis of large sample groups?	Yes	No
Can identify foods with (acceptable) traces of gluten from absolutely gluten-free foods?	Yes	Yes
Can discriminate foods above and below current codes for gluten threshold?	Yes	Yes
Cost per test?	Few dollars US	Few dollars US
Tests per kit?	41-44 duplicate	8-10 tests

The gluten home test represents a whole new concept in consumer capabilities. It represents the first test for use by "lay" individuals who are allergic or intolerant to a specific food group or food constituent which enables them to test the foods they eat. Quite conceivably, antibody-based tests for soya and milk proteins, lectin-binding tests for galactose or antibody tests for food colourings and preservatives could be modified for use in the home. However, correct and appropriate interpretation of results will be critical.

REFERENCES

1 Dissanayake AS, Truelove SC, Whitehead R.Lack of harmful effect of oats on small-intestinal mucosa in coeliac disease. Brit Med J 1974;4:189-191.

2 Anand BS, Piris J, Truelove SC. The role of various cereals in coeliac disease. Quart J Med 1978;47:101-110.

3 Zareba J. Detection of gliadin in gluten-free bread by means of double diffusion on agar gel. Pol Tyg Lek 1968;23:1962-1963.

4 Keyser JW, Mahler RF. Detection of gluten in flour. Lancet i 1968;678.

5 Lietze A. Quantitation of food adulterants by multiple radial immunodiffusion. II. Wheat in bread sold as "wheat free" for the use of allergy patients. J Assoc Off Anal Chem 1969;52:988-995.

6 Guenther HO.Detection of plant proteins in meat products. I. Methods and results of routine work. Ann Nutr Aliment 1977;31:179-181.

7 Baudner S. Immunological food analysis. Definitions, methods, examples from cereal research. Getreide Mehl und Brot 1978;32:330-333.

8 Kaczkowski J, Jurowska E, Moskal M. Immunological method of wheat gluten detection in food products designed for coeliac disease patients. Acta Aliment Polonica 1987;11:177-183.
9 Bauer F, Stachelberger H.Immunoelectrophoretic analysis of non-meat protein in meat products. II. Counter current electrophoresis of wheat gluten (gliadin). Chem Microbiol Technol Lebensm 1988;11:132-136.
10 Ciclitira PJ, Lennox ES. A radioimmunoassay for alpha- and beta-gliadins. Clin Sci 1983;64:655-659.
11 Windemann H, Fritschy F, Baumgartner E. Enzyme linked immunosorbent assay for wheat alpha-gliadin and whole gliadin. Biochim Biophys Acta 1982;709:110-121.
12 Fritschy F, Winderman H, Baumgartner E, Quantitative determination of wheat gliadins in foods by enzyme-linked immunosorbent assay. Z Lebems Unters Forsch. 1985; 181: 379-385.
13 Troncone R, Vitale M, Donantiello A, Farris E, Rossi G, Auricchio S. A sandwich enzyme immunoassay for wheat gliadin. J Immunol Methods 1986;92:21-23.
14 Freedman AR, Galfre G, Gal E, Ellis MJ, Ciclitira PJ. Monoclonal antibody ELISA to quantitate wheat gliadin contamination of gluten-free foods. J Immunol Methods 1987;98:123-127.
15 Ayob MK, Rittenburg J. Allen JC, Smith CJ. Development of a rapid enzyme-linked immunosorbent assay (ELISA) for gliadin determination in food. Food Hydrocolloids 1988;2:39-49.
16 Cooke WT, Holmes GKT. Coeliac Disease. Churchill Livingstone. Edinburgh.
17 Cole SG, Kagnoff MF. Coeliac Disease. Annu Rev Nutr 1985;5:241-266.
18 Meier P, Windemann H, Baumgartner E. Determination of the alpha-gliadin content of heated foods containing gluten or being "gluten-free". Z Lebens Unters Forsch 1984;178:361-365.
19 Skerritt JH, Smith RA. A sensitive monoclonal antibody based test for gluten detection. Studies with cooked or processed foods. J Sci Food Agric 1985;36:980-985.
20 Heppell LMJ, Cant AJ, Kilshaw PJ. Reduction in the antigenicity of whey proteins by heat treatments: a possible strategy for producing a hypoallergenic infant milk formule. Brit J Nutr 1984;51:29-36.
21 Skerritt JH, Smith RA, Wrigley CW, Underwood PA. Monoclonal antibodies to gliadin proteins used to examine cereal grain protein homologies. J Cereal Sci 1984;2:215-224.
22 Skerritt JH, Lew PY. Homologies between grain storage of different cereals. I. Monoclonal antibody reaction with total protein extracts. J Cereal Sci 1990;11:103-121.
23 Skerritt JH. A sensitive monoclonal antibody based assy for gluten detection. Quantitative immunoassay. J Sci Food Agric 1985;36:987-994.
24 Skerritt JH. Detection and quantitation of cereal protein in foods using specific anzyme-linked monoclonal antibodies. Food Technol Aust 1985;37:570-572.
25 Skerritt JH, Martinuzzi O. Effects of solid phase and antigen solvent on the binding and immunoassay of water-insoluble flour proteins. J Immunol Methods 1986;88:217-224.
26 Freedman AR, Galfre G, Gal E, Ellis HJ. Detection of wheat gliadin contamination of gluten free foods by monoclonal antibody dot-immunobinding assay. Clin Chim Acta 1987;166:323-328.

GLUTEN-FREE PRODUCTS, THE DUTCH EXPERIENCE.

F.W. Janssen, G.H. Hägele, J.A. de Baaij. Inspectorate of Public Health, Regional Food Inspection Service, PO Box 9012, 7200 GN, Zutphen, The Netherlands.

Interest from our Food Inspection Services in gluten free food has been latent for a long time and it is only recently that we became interested again in analyzing "gluten free" food for its residual gluten content. Our investigations departed as a spin-off from another area, a project on the detection of non-meat proteins (casein, soy protein, whey and gluten) in meat products. Though we found that the incorporation of wheat gluten in these products is not yet a current practice, presumably by consequence of its poor functional properties, we noticed to our surprise that a number of meat products had been labeled as to contain starch, while in fact wheat flour had been used. Such mis-labelling can result in gluten levels of up to 1% in these products, which could be considered suitable for inclusion in a gluten free diet, as judged from the label. These findings triggered a general interest in the composition of "gluten free" foods and in addition to meat products we determined the gluten content of many products, either labeled as "gluten free" or supposed to be naturally gluten free. We used ELISA or dot blot assay to screen these products and confirmed the presence of gluten by performing a more extended analysis by SDS electrophoresis, blotting and immunochemical staining of protein (gliadin) bands. Detection limit with the latter method was 1 mg gliadin/100 g product. Miscellaneous results were obtained with products based on wheat starch. In 80% of the wheat starch based bread mixes we could detect gliadin. Levels varied from 10-100 mg/100g. In all samples of bread which had been baked from these flours, gliadin could be determined. Some levels were higher than calculated, indicating contamination with wheat flour. In a custard powder based on wheat starch we found even 275 mg/100 g. Though one might consider the presence of residual gliadin in wheat starch by consequence a general phenomenon, this is not the case. The few exceptions on the contrary demonstrate that wheat starch can be prepared which contains less than 1 mg/100 g. These results question whether some producers of "gluten free" starches are working according to the current state of the art. Another problem is posed by contamination of products which are naturally gluten free. In a set of 28 samples of flour (rice, buckwheat, maize, millet) which were not labeled as "gluten free", we found two severely contaminated buckwheat flours (200, resp 300 mg gliadin/100 g) and one mixed flour (buckwheat, rice and millet) containing 275 mg gliadin/100 g. This constitutes an average contamination incidence of about 10%. No contamination with gluten could be detected in composite products labeled as "gluten free" which were prepared from rice, maize or millet flour.

INTRODUCTION

In the Netherlands it is the task of the Inspectorate for Health Protection to enforce and promote compliance with regulations pertaining to goods, as laid down in several food laws and regulations. The aforementioned Inspectorate (850 employees) is an executive department of the Ministry of Welfare, Public Health and

M. L. Mearin and C. J. J. Mulder (eds.), Coeliac Disease, 95–100.

Cultural Affairs. There are 13 Regional Inspectorates, each with trained staff and a well equipped laboratory.
Although each laboratory is carrying out regular daily investigational work, i.e. microbiological and chemical examination of foodstuffs and commodities, each of them has a dedicated field of interest, a group of products which receives special attention. For a number of years one of the fields of interest of the Regional Inspectorate Zutphen has been meat and meat products and proteins for food application. It is this special interest in protein analysis and the expertise which we acquired with regard to electrophoresis and immunoassays which made our laboratory to take the lead within the Inspectorate to investigate gluten free food for gliadin content. The interest in gluten free food had become dormant within the Inspectorate some years ago and it was just recently that an active interest in examining gluten free foods for residual gluten content became stirred up again. Our interests in gluten free products started as a spin-off from a quite different area, a project on the detection of non-meat proteins (casein, soy protein, whey and wheat gluten) in meat products.
This work aroused a general interest with regard to the presence of gluten in other foods as well. We determine the gluten content in a number of gluten free products next to meat products.

Sources of unintentional gluten intake by patients with coeliac disease (CD), can be classified as follows:

A Residual gluten in gluten free wheat starch used for bread mixes.
B Contamination of foods which are "naturally" gluten free, e.g. rice or maize flours with wheat flour.
C Mis-labelling of foods in which gluten is present but which do not have any gluten containing constituents in the ingredient list.
D Consumption of products with respect to which no unambiguous scientific opinion exists as to whether they are toxic to coeliacs. An example is beer. Though some consider the drinking of beer safe, others have a different view (1).

STUDIED SOURCES OF UNINTENTIONAL GLUTEN INTAKE

CATEGORY A

Very miscellaneous results were obtained with products based on wheat starch. In 80 % of the wheat starch based bread mixes we could detect gliadin (detection level 1 mg/100 g). Levels found varied from 10-100 mg/100g. In all samples of bread which had been baked from these flours, gliadin could be determined. Some levels were higher than calculated, indicating contamination with wheat flour. In a custard powder based on wheat starch we found even 275 mg/100 g. Though one might consider the presence of residual gliadin in wheat starch by consequence a general phenomenon, this is not the case. The few exceptions illustrate the fact that wheat starch can be prepared containing less than 1 mg/100 g gliadin. These results make it questionable whether some producers of wheat starches are working conform to the current state of the art in gluten free wheat starch production.

CATEGORY B

Another problem is posed by contamination of products which are naturally gluten free. In a set of 28 samples of various flours (rice, buckwheat, maize, millet) which were not labelled as "gluten free", we found two severely contaminated buckwheat flours (200, resp. 300 mg gliadin/100 g) and one mixed flour (buckwheat, rice and millet) containing 275 mg gliadin/100 g. This constitutes an average contamination incidence of about 10%. On the contrary no contamination with gluten could be detected in composite products labeled as "gluten free" which were prepared from rice, maize or millet flour.

CATEGORY C

As stated above it was our work on the determination of wheat gluten in meat products which initiated our interest in gluten free foods. Though we found that the incorporation of wheat gluten in these products is not yet current practice, presumably by consequence of its poor functional properties, we noticed to our surprise that a number of meat products had been labelled as to contain starch, while in fact wheat flour had been used. Such mis-labelling could result in gluten levels of up to 1% in meat products, which could be considered (as judged from the label) as suitable for inclusion in a gluten free diet. The examination of meat products with respect to the presence of the aforementioned nonmeat proteins is now carried out routinely and many more producers have been found to neglect labelling requirements with respect to gluten. Upon questioning the reasons for negligence they proved to be almost ignorant with respect to the impact of such mis-labelling for CD patients. Some even objected that to most consumers "starch" was a more informative ingredient statement than "wheat flour"!

CATEGORY D

Very conflicting opinions have been reported with respect to the consumption of beer. Some Coeliac Societies (though not really promoting drinking beer) have adopted a rather liberal attitude. In one of the literary digests in our national Coeliac News Quarterly a report from our Belgian colleagues was quoted, who found no hordein in several brands of Belgian beer. In contrast with this Ciclitira (1) reports that malt based beer contained up to 6 mg/pint, an amount which he considers high enough to exacerbate symptoms in susceptible individuals. We analysed 22 brands of Dutch, German and Belgian beer with SDS electrophoresis, blotting and immunoperoxidase staining. Though we did not observe a distinct band pattern, the dense and heavily stained smears indicated the presence of gliadin-like immunoreactive material with a mol size comparable to that of hordeïn in some brands. Very dense smears were observed with some Belgian beers (Gueuze beers), in which barley had been partly substituted by wheat. Some other brands, notably the low alcohol ones showed on the contrary completely void lanes. These results confirm Ciclitiras findings that hordeïn is present in many brands of beer. We do not endorse the conclusion that those beers which do not show immunoreactive material are safe to drink by CD patients. In these beers low molecular peptide fragments with the ability to exacerbate symptoms may still be present. Work is in progress to find out whether results obtained with sandwich ELISA's support our findings.

LEGISLATION

One of the most discouraging aspects of analyzing "gluten free foods" for gluten content is that the legal framework for these products is inadequate and vague. The Dutch "Decree on the Labelling of Dietary Foods" demands that food for special (dietary) nutrition must be either prepared to be suitable, or be "naturally" suitable to the purposed dietary need. No limiting gliadin content is however explicitly stated in any Dutch food legislation. This defect and the rather liberal limiting gliadin content mentioned in the Codex Alimentarius Recommendations of 1981 (although not explicitly adopted in Dutch legislation) makes it extremely difficult to exert remedial action on producers. Within the Inspectorate the prevailing opinion is that foods labelled as "gluten free" should comply to a zero level of gliadin. Laws of precedents are lacking however. One of the most promising feasibilities is perhaps that our "Decree on the Labelling of Dietary Foods" requires that the amount of gluten which is actually present has to be stated on the label of all pre-packed "gluten free" foods. Due to the fact that the introduction of reliable analytical techniques like ELISA for this purpose is of a quite recent date and that (though work on collaborative trials is in progress) no results with respect to reproducibility and validity are known, it is perhaps not yet expedient to enforce this labelling requirement.

ANALYTICAL ASPECTS

In a litigious society we have to be sure that the results of our analysis comply with the highest qualitative and quantitative standards. We must realize that we are often working on analyses which are present in complex matrices, the composition of which may vary to a great extent and will be as a rule unknown to the analyst. In our laboratory we therefore adopted - at least for the time being - a two stage procedure.

First we determine or detect gluten by a sandwich ELISA or cost effective dot blot procedure. If gluten is present we confirm the results by SDS electrophoresis, blotting and immunochemical staining of the gliadin bands (2). It is on purpose that we are using SDS electrophoresis and not the common standard (ISTA) acid PAGE (3). The latter has been designed to maximize within-species variability and is suitable to identify cultivars. Expression of polymorphy in our electropherograms hampers a correct identification at the species level and it would also be more difficult to distinguish specific from unspecific staining. But even when performing the analysis with this elaborate procedure the analysis may be flawed: if the protein pattern cannot be matched to one of the patterns of our reference bank, we do not know whether this constitutes a false positive result, the presence of a wheat variety unknown to us or the use of modified gluten.

So far however, an extensive majority of positive samples can be classified as to contain wheat, rye or barley, while only a minor part proves to be unclassifiable.

Despite the fact that the analysis by consequence is getting rather complicated, we have adopted this procedure as a provisional standard. The most important rationale to do so, is that a result obtained with an ELISA procedure which in the end turns

out as false positive will jeopardize the confidence of legal authorities in the analytical possibilities. We expect that in due course, experience growing, this confirmation will prove to be superfluous. In fact we strongly advocate the use of sandwich ELISA's as a first line approach. One of the most favourable aspects of sandwich ELISA's over e.g. dotblot assays is that the signal which we always obtain in the latter with rice, maize, sorghum and millet is suppressed to a great extent.
This is a phenomenon which we quite often observe: sandwich ELISA's are more discriminative than dot blot.

SEVERAL MECHANISMS MAY BE OPERATIVE:

1 One might assume that polyclonal antibodies prepared with denatured gliadin as immunogen and absorbed in an homogeneous phase with native cross-reacting prolamins from e.g. millet, sorghum or rice, might still give cross-reaction with denatured prolamins from these species. A condition would be that these "denatured" or "interior" epitopes become exposed on the binding of the protein to nitrocellulose and are not exposed in e.g. a sandwich type assay.

2 The aforementioned hypothesis cannot explain the cross-reactivity of monoclonal antibodies, observed using dot blot assays, unless we assume that some relevant epitopes are shared by wheat, millet, maize etc., but are surface oriented in case of wheat and are hidden (yet becoming exposed on absorption on nitrocellulose) in case of millet etc.

3 The most probable cause of the enhanced discriminating power of a sandwich ELISA vs e.g. dotblotting on nitrocellulose might however be that in the former case a number of epitopes are actually "consumed" upon binding of the antigen to the wall-coated antibody. If one assumes that the epitopes with the highest affinity are preferentially bound during the first step of the ELISA by the wall-coated antibody, such enhanced selectivity of a sandwich type of immunoassay becomes quite comprehensable.

CONCLUSIONS

There are several potential causes of unintentional gluten intake by CD patients: wheat starch based bread mixes, contaminated flours, mis-labelled food products etc. As judged from our market survey it becomes manifest that all categories may in fact contribute to the gluten intake. Though the relative importance of each category is not known, one of our future goals must be to eliminate these causes. A more active propagation of information about CD among food producers would in our opinion be one of the best means to achieve this goal.
In The Netherlands, like in many other countries, extensive lists of foods are available which are suitable in a gluten free diet. There is no guarantee for completeness and validity of these lists as all contributions (new entries, deletions and changes) are voluntary. A general awareness among producers should be promoted to keep these lists updated. Due to the voluntary character of this system any

repressive action from the side of the Inspectorate for Health Protection with respect to the validity of these lists has to be avoided. Legislation with regard to the categories mentioned above is defect or vague, which impedes remedial actions by the aforementioned Inspectorate to a great extent.

The good news is that analytical possibilities are rapidly improving. The procedure of analysis as adopted by us warrants that no "false positive" results will be obtained. We expect that the confirmation of the results with SDS-electrophoresis, blotting and immunochemical detection of gliadin wil become redundant in the near future. If results of collaborative trials are satisfying we will be able to effectuate the requirement of our "Decree on the Labelling of Dietary Foods" that the amount of gluten must be declared. Scientific agreement about the permissive level of gluten in foods labelled as "gluten free" and implementation of this level in national or EEC legislation will then rule out existing obscurities.

REFERENCES

1 Ciclitira PJ, Analytical methods and clinical effects of small quantities of gluten in food for Celiacs. Rome, 26-11-1989.

2 Janssen FW, Voortman G, de Baaij JA. Detection of Wheat Gluten, Whey Protein, Casein, Ovalbumin and Soy Protein in Heated Meat Products by Electrophoresis, Blotting and Immunoperoxidase Staining. J of Agriculture and Food Chemistry 1987;35:563-567.

3 Cooper SR. Report of the Rules Committee. Seed Science and Technology 1987;15:555-575.

THE QUEST FOR GLIADIN: LIMITS AND TOLERANCE.

W.Th.J.M. Hekkens, Dept of Physiology, University of Leiden, Duinwetering 27, 2203 LH, Noordwijk, The Netherlands.

Limits of "gliadin" in the diet of gluten-sensitive patients can be considered from different points of view. It is not only gliadin that is toxic to these patients but also, as we know from the work of Dicke, Weyers and van de Kamer, rye and barley. Hansted found that also oats was toxic, be it to a lesser extend. Elimination of these products as such does not garantee that a food is "gluten free". Contamination during transport, milling or processing can happen easily and stresses the need of good analytical methods to determine the extend of contamination. Gliadin - or rather the prolamins from wheat, rye, barley and oats - can be altered in structure by hydrolysis and heat denaturation; two processes that are used extensively in industry to alter the physico-chemical properties of the prolamins for use in a great array of products. As immunochemical methods are used for their determination, one must be aware of all these factors. Apart from the analytical problems in the determination of prolamins, there is the question of the amount of prolamin a patient can tolerate. We can distinguish three different actions of gliadin. First there is an allergic reaction in individuals allergic to it. Although this is not necessarily gluten-sensitivity in the classical way, a number of persons have immediate adverse reactions; the level of tolerance is almost zero. In real gluten-sensitive enteropathy, the level of tolerance is higher. There are indications that an average of 10 mg per day can be tolerated over a long period of time without detectable damage of the intestinal lining. As we know from epidemiologic studies on gluten-sensitive patients on a normal diet, the risk for intestinal malignancies is increased as compared to patients on a "gluten-free" diet. There is no study comparing patients using an absolutely gluten-free diet with patients having the conventional gluten-free diet that will always contain a low amount of prolamin by contamination. Therefore the long-term effect of a diet with a low gluten content is still open to discussion.

INTRODUCTION

Toxicity of a substance, no matter if it is toxic to the whole population or to a specific group, is not only a matter of the character of the molecule, but also a matter of concentration. The character of the gliadin molecule has been discussed in many papers that appeared in the last 40 years, after the discovery by Dicke, Weijers and van de Kamer (1) that it was the alcohol-soluble part of the wheat protein that causes the damaging effect on the intestinal lining in patients with Coeliac Disease (CD). Toxicity can be intrinsic, meaning that a molecule as such is the toxic substance, or can be extrinsic meaning that the molecule is only toxic after metabolic conversion inside the body. Apart from the fact, already published in 1958 by Frazer (2) that the toxicity of gliadin remains after peptic-tryptic-pancreatic digestion of the protein, one can say that a peptide formed during that digestion is the intrinsic toxic factor in CD. The problem is that we do not know what exactly is that peptide, not its minimal chain lenght, nor its amino acid sequence. We know

M. L. Mearin and C. J. J. Mulder (eds.), Coeliac Disease, 101–106.

however that this sequence is not only found in the prolamins from wheat, but also in that of rye, barley and oats. We even could postulate that there is more than one peptide sequence that contains the toxic principle.
The concentration of a toxic substance is also something that we have to discuss. In the Codex Alimentarius Standard for "Gluten-free" foods, as proposed in 1981, the definition of "gluten-free" is based on the nitrogen content of the gluten-containing cereal grains. Accepting that nitrogen content of 0.05 g per 100 grammes of these grains on dry matter basis, means the acceptance of roughly 100 mg of gliadin per 100 grammes of dry product derived from cereal grains. Table I gives an indication of the "prolamin" content of the different cereal grains.

TABLE I PROTEIN AND PROLAMIN CONTENT OF THE CEREAL GRAINS

Cereal	Prolamin	Protein in %	Prolamin in%
wheat	gliadin	10 - 15	4 - 7.5
rye	secalin	9 - 14	3 - 7
barley	hordein	10 - 14	3.5 - 7
oats	avenin	8 - 14	0.8 - 2.1
maize	zein	7 - 13	3.5 - 7

Translated into the Codex limits one can say that an intake of not more than 1.3 gram of pure wheat grains or flour meets the amount as allowed by this standard. The problem however is that the standard speaks of the amount contained in a food and not of the amount of that food that can be taken by a person who is sensitive to it. The standard speaks of limits, not of tolerance.

THE GLUTEN-FREE FOOD

When we accept the ELISA-technique for the determination of prolamins in food, then the question arises, what are we really measuring? The working group of prolamin analysis and toxicity that I founded in 1985 studied this question together with a new proposal to add an analytical technique to the draft of the Codex Standard. In principle there are two possibilities to perform the ELISA-determination. A polyclonal antibody, made against a whole gliadin, or a monoclonal antibody reacting with only one epitope in the mixture of prolamins can be used in the determination. The advantage of a polyclonal is that more than one epitope in the total amount of gliadin molecules is determined and the risk of variability in the determination of different grain varieties is greatly reduced. The advantage of a monoclonal antibody is its reproducibility in production, especially when great quantities are necessary. Both methods however need a standard to be reproducible as the titer of all antibodies changes with time. Here again a choice must be made. We have chosen for a standard, made by alcoholic extraction of vital gluten and lyophylisation of the extract. In this way we include as many epitopes as possible and this allows the comparison of results obtained by groups using an antibody raised against a different variety of wheat. From the Codex Standard one could get the impression that the analysis of food is only necessary when ingredients derived from wheat, rye, barley or oats are used. We know however that also in other cases it is possible to find higher or lower quantities of prolamins in the food. There are a number of posibilities for contamination of the end product. Table II summarizes the most important of them.

TABLE II POSSIBLE WAYS OF FOOD CONTAMINATION WITH PROLAMINS

Crop contamination
Storage
Transport
Milling
Manufacturing

We have seen in several cases a contamination of up to 5% of presumebly non-toxic grains by wheat or rye, so if a contamination is possible, it is worthwile to determine the gliadin content in the end product.

PROLAMIN HEATING AND COOKING

The determination of gliadin is based on crude, native gliadin and the patient mostly uses products that are heated or cooked. It depends on the method chosen what the influence of these processes is on the results of the determination. Meier (3) heated gliadin at different temperatures and determined the outcome on the determination with a polyclonal antibody. He found a substantial reduction in quantity after heating. At a temperature of 90°C, only 10% of the gliadin was recovered by the assay. Skerrit (4) however claims that his method, using a monoclonal antibody against the more heat-stable omega-gliadin could determine 100% of the gliadin in cooked water-gliadin suspensions but also only 5% in cooked water-flour suspensions. Confirmation of his results could be of great help in the near future.

PROLAMIN DEGRADATION

Digestion of gliadin has two aspects. Apart from a possible change in toxicity, the chain lenght has an effect on the determination by an ELISA-technique. No good study on these effects is available to my knowledge. In our own experience a peptic-tryptic digest of gliadin could not be determined with our polyclonal antibody. A solution of this digest does not inhibit the determination of whole gliadin, when added to the extract in the determination. No experiments of this kind are performed with a monoclonal antibody-based assay. The determination of degraded products is important as there are many products that for technological reasons contain partly hydrolysed gluten. Also in some brands of beer there are peptides that possibly are toxic to patients with CD and that escape determination at this moment.

OTHER PROLAMINS

The prolamins of rye, barley and oats are also toxic to patients with CD. They give a crossreaction with an antiserum against gliadin. This means that there are epitopes in these prolamins that are shared. This makes it possible to use the antigliadin antiserum also for the determination of secalin, hordein and avenin. Skerrit (5,6) found that his antibody also reacts with secalin and hordein. It does not react with avenin however. Apart from that, a number of these antibodies produced and used by different authors crossreact also with zein. A positive reaction thus can be a false positive and in that case a confirmation of the presence or absence of a toxic prolamin is necessary. This can be done by a blotting technique or by HPLC.

DETECTION LIMITS

In all the methods published so far (6,8), the limits of detection is of the same order. About 15 nanogram per gram of dry product can be determined. This is 1.5 mg per 100 grammes and is far within the limit of 100 mg as comes from the nitrogen-content based previous method. The limit of detection of course is not the limit of tolerance.

LIMITS OF TOLERANCE

If we know how much prolamin is in our food, then the next question is how much can we tolerate. The absolute absence of prolamins in our food is something that we can aim at, but in practice it is extremely difficult to achieve. Small amounts of gliadin can have different effects, depending on the condition of the patient and the duration of the intake and eventual previous periods of exposure to the toxic prolamins. There is one group of patients that is sensitive to very small amounts; they are not the patients with CD but they have an allergic reaction to wheat, especially wheat prolamin. The reaction is an immediate one, as is the recovery after elimination of the agent. Apart from that group there is the group of real coeliacs where an intestinal lesion is the primary effect of the intake of toxic prolamins. One could ask if it is necessary for them to avoid all toxic prolamins or if the intestine can tolerate small amounts. There have been very little studies in this direction. Ciclitira (9) has challenged patients over a period of six weeks with an average daily amount of 1.8 mg of gliadin. After that period, he found that some of them had signs of diarrhea but no other symptoms indicating an intestinal damage was observed. Ejderhamn (10) has studied children for a longer period of time. He followed 8 children with CD over 8-14 years. The calculated mean daily intake of gliadin was 7 mg, the average age of the children was 15 years. When small intestinal biopsies were taken after that period there was no evidence of mucosal damage in these patients. This means that in these children no direct effect was seen by an intake of roughly less than 10 mg of gliadin per day.

We could analyse the effect of small amounts of gliadin in one of the patients in Dr Mearin's clinic. She had a patient with a proven CD that did well on a gluten-free breadmix (A) in the clinic as well as at home. After some time the child got

symptoms of the disease again. Hospitalisation did not improve her symptoms and after some improvement on prednison, she was sent home. Here her mother realised that she had changed from one gluten-free breadmix to another (B) and she decided to return to the old mix again. This gave the improvement that was not obtained in the clinic. As the mother and the clinic still had some material of the different batches used, we were able to analyse them, together with other samples (B-1,B-2,B-3) of the same breadmix. The results are given in table III.
As can be seen from the table both an earlier mix as well as two later ones had a level well under the mix that caused the damage. Calculating back the amount of gliadin that the child had ingested during that period, learned us that she got between 14 and 28 mg gliadin per day when on the breadmix B and between 5 and 10 mg on mix A. Although the period of consumption was much shorter than in the Ejderhamn study, it is of interest to see that the intake without damage is of the same order. This could mean that the intestine in capable to handle small amounts of gliadin without a risk of damage. The limit of tolerance being 10 mg per day. This observation on the other hand demonstrates that a regular control of the different batches of a product is necessary to stay within the levels of safety.

TABLE III ELISA-ANALYSIS OF BREAD-MIXES USED BY A PATIENT WITH CD

Sample code	Batch date		Gliadin in mg/100 gram
A	july	'88	8
B	october	'88	25
B-1	july	'88	3
B-2	februari	'89	7
B-3	februari	'89	3

Based on these figures for tolerance, we consider a level of less than 10 mg of gliadin per 100 grammes dry product derived from cereal grains as safe to coeliac patients, provided that the intake per day is not more than 100 grammes of that flour. Apart from the direct effect on the intestinal wall, prolamins have also an effect on malignancy in coeliac patients. We know from many theoretical studies that the effect of initiation in malignancy is a cumulative effect. This could mean that even a small amount of gluten in the long run increases the risk of malignancy. This could also be the case with gliadin, unless the intestinal wall can render the small amount of gliadin presented to it non-toxic before it reaches the enterocyte. There are indications that this is the case. Holmes (11) compared the incidence of malignancy in patients with CD on a "gluten-free" diet, on a gluten-reduced diet and on a gluten-containing diet. They found that the risk was increased for those on a gluten-reduced and a gluten-containing diet, but not for those on a "gluten-free" diet as compared with the normal population. In my opinion we can safely take it for granted that the "gluten-free" diet used by these patients was not absolutely gluten-free. When we accept that, we see that also in terms of malignancy the small intestine of coeliac patients has not lost all his capacity to defend itself against small amounts of potentially toxic substances presented to it and an intake of maximally 10 mg of gliadin per day - as indicated already - can be taken as safe also in this respect.

TOXICITY AND IMMUNOGENICITY

By accepting the methods described, for the determination of prolamins in the "gluten-free" diet of coeliac patients, we must realize that the epitopes that are picked up by the antibodies in the assay, are not necessarily the same as the peptide sequences that cause the toxic reaction in coeliac patients. We do not determine toxicity, but prove the presence or absence of prolamins in general, the toxic fragments included. As long as the real toxic fragment is not known, this general method is the only basis for a reliable analysis.

REFERENCES

1 Dicke WK, Weijers HA, van de Kamer JH. An investigation into the injurious constituents of wheat in connection with their action on patients with coeliac disease. Acta Paediatr 1953;42:223-231.

2 Frazer AC, Fletcher F, Ross C, Shaw B, Sammons HG, Schneider R. Gluten-induced enteropathy. The effect of partially digested gluten. Lancet 1958;2:252-255.

3 Meier P, Windemann H, Baumgartner E. Determination of alpha-gliadin content of heated food, containing and free of gluten. Z. Lebensm Unters Forsch 1984;178:361-365.

4 Skerritt JH, Smith RA. A sensitive monoclonal-antibody-based test for gluten detection: studies with cooked or processed foods. J Sci Food Agric 1985;36:980-986.

5 Skerritt JH. A sensitive monoclonal-antibody-based test for gluten detection: quantitative immunoassay. J Sci Food Agric 1985;36:987-994.

6 Skerritt JH, Diment JA, Wrigley CW. A sensitive monoclonal-antibody-based test for gluten detection: choice of primary and secondary antibodies. J Sci Food Agr 1985;36:995-1003.

7 Troncone R, Vitale M, Donatiello A, Faris E, Rossi G, Auricchio S. A sandwich enzyme immunoassay for wheat gliadin. J Imm Methods 1986;92:21-23.

8 McKillop DF, Gosling JP, Stevens FM, Fottrell PF. Enzyme immunoassay of gliadin in food. Biochem Soc Trans 1985;13:486-487.

9 Ciclitira PJ, Cerio R, Ellis HJ, Maxton D, Nelufer JM, McCartney JM. Evaluation of a gliadin-containing gluten-free product in coeliac disease. Hum Nutr: Clin Nutr 1985;39c:303-308.

10 Ejderhamn J, Veress B, Strandvik B. The long term effect of continual ingestion of wheat starch containing gluten-free products in coeliac patients. Proc Fourth Intern Symp on Coeliac Disease, London 1988; In press.

11 Holmes GKT, Prior P, Lane MR, Pope D, Allan RN. Malignancy in coeliac disease - effect of a gluten free diet. Gut 1989;30:333.

THE INCIDENCE OF COELIAC DISEASE AND CHANGES IN GLUTEN CONSUMPTION.

B. Kristiansson, H. Ascher, I. Odenman, L. Sandberg*. Dep. of Pediatrics, University of Gothenburg, Götenborg, Sweden. * The Regional Blood Centre, Sahlgrenska Hospital, Götenborg, Sweden.

Changes in frequency of childhood coeliac disease (CD) were studied retrospectively among children born in the city of Göteborg, Sweden, between 1970 and 1988. Altogether 183 patients with CD were found. Seventy percent were verified according to the ESPGAN criteria. Eighty-three percent were below two years at the first small intestinal biopsy. There was a significant increase of CD during the study period. This increase appeared to be continuous with a relatively sharp rise to a higher basal level for birth cohorts of 1982 and later.
The number of cases of CD per 1 000 liveborn infants increased threefold from 0.98 to 3.07 ($p = 0.0004$) with a mean difference of 1.31 ± 0.59 (99.9% confidence limit) between children born before and after 1982. The following factors have been studied in order to find the cause of the increased incidence of CD: duration of breastfeeding, the age at introduction of cow's milk and gluten into the diet, potential changes of the amount of gluten consumed and HLA antigens of the children. The duration of breastfeeding increased significantly during the observation period, as did the age when foods containing cow's milk and gluten were introduced. The amount of gluten consumed, as assessed by four-day records, indicate that infants now consume approximately 1.5 times more gluten at the age of 12 months, and 1.1 times more at the age of 18 months compared to the seventies.
There was no difference in prevalence of various HLA antigens, known to be associated with CD. The increase could be explained by at least two different factors.
The first one is the increased amount of gluten consumed by Swedish infants and young children. The increased consumption of gluten is basically caused by the industrial baby foods, which, due to the industrial processing resulted in a close to doubled increase of gluten in the most common industrial baby foods used (gruel and porridge).
The second factor is the increasing awareness about the disease and its cause among both physicians and laymen, resulting in wider indications for small intestinal biopsies, also at modest symptoms of gastrointestinal disease and growth deviation. This is reflected in an over all improved weight for age at the time of the first intestinal biopsy. The increase in frequency of CD is the first reported in twenty years and makes CD one of the most common chronic diseases in Swedish children.

INTRODUCTION

Decreasing frequency of CD has been reported from several places in the United Kingdom and Ireland (1-3). Several reports of them had the title "CD is disappearing!". From Finland a changing pattern was reported with a decreasing frequency of CD in young infants and children and possibly increasing frequency in older age goups (4). From Italy one paper on unchanged frequency was recently published (5). The factors responsible for the changes observed have been related to

M. L. Mearin and C. J. J. Mulder (eds.), Coeliac Disease, 107–114.

changes in feeding patterns of young children. The duration of breast-feeding, the age at introduction of cow's milk and gluten proteins have been particularly studied, as well as the impact of infections such as that of adenovirus type 12 (6). There has been no unequivocal explanation for the findings reported.

PATIENTS AND METHODS

We have had the opportunity to study the frequency of childhood CD in Gothenburg, a city with 430.000 inhabitants, during the last 20 year, and to relate the findings to potentially relevant factors. All cases of CD in children born in the city of Gothenburg between 1970 and 1988 were included. The number of patients with CD in each annual birth cohort was calculated as birth prevalence rate (BPR), expressed per 1000 live births. By calculating BPR fot three cohorts, moving three-year averages of BPR were determined. The cumulated incidence of CD was calculated as the number of CD diagnosed before the age of two years in each birth cohort, expressed per 1000 live birth. HLA antigens were analysed in two representative samples of children with CD: 30 children from the seventies and 30 from the late eighties. HLA typing (ABC- and DR) was performed at the tissue typing department. Another representative sample of 40 children (20 with CD and 20 without) investigated during the late eighties were analysed with neutralizing tests against adenovirus 12 antibodies. To estimate the amount of gluten consumed in the population 4 day records of dietary intake were collected from four groups of children. Healthy and hospital selected controls of age 12 and 18 months were compared. There were 10 children in each group. The calculations on the prolamin contents of the foods consumed were based on information obtained from the baby food industry. The prolamin contents of the proteins of the grains was estimated at 45% for wheat, 40% for rye, 40% for barley and 10% for oats. The following factors were analysed: duration of breast-feeding, age at introduction of gluten and of cow's milk protein, duration of mixed-feeding (combined breast and cow's milk or gluten), changes of the quantity of gluten consumed, the occurrence of antibodies to adenovirus 12 and HLA antigens.

RESULTS

A total of 184 children with CD were included in the study. The number of children diagnosed as CD has steadily increased ($p<0.001$) throughout the study period, see Figure 1. On an average there were 5-6 new cases of CD annually in the first half of the study period, increasing to the double from around 1983 and to three times more at the end. The black bars indicate children with an age < 2 years at the time of the first intestinal biopsy, and it is seen that this category is also increasing ($p<0.001$). BPR, the birth prevalence rate, indicates the frequency of CD related to the population basis for each birth cohort (Table I). BPR increased significantly throughout the study period ($p<0.001$). Calculated as a rolling 3 year average it increased from approximately 1 to almost 3/1000 over the period. In a strictly epidemiological sense the BPR has the weakness to give longer chances for the older cohorts to acquire the diagnosis compared to the younger ones. This is adjusted for by calculating the cumulated incidence of CD diagnosed before the age of 2 years for each cohort (Figure 2). Again, the cumulated incidence has clearly and significantly increased (=0.79, p=0.0001).

FIGURE I

NEW CASES OF CHILDHOOD CD BY AGE, GROUP AND YEAR.

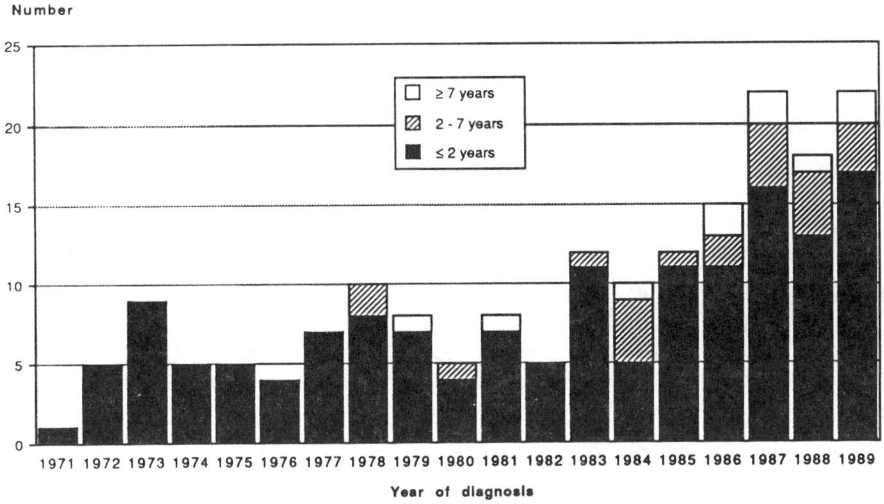

FIGURE II

CUMULATED INCIDENCE OF CD IN CHILDREN <2 YEARS OF AGE, BY BIRTH COHORT

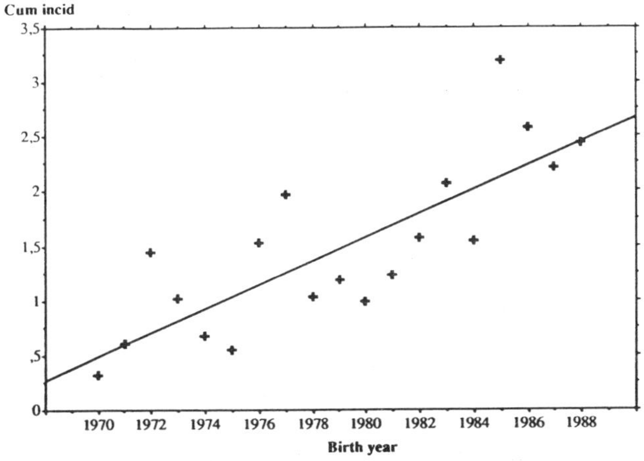

WHICH ARE THE REASONS FOR THIS OBSERVED INCREASE?

The most immediate thoughts were factors related to feeding patterns of infants and young children. Had there been any major changes in this respect during the observation period? In children with CD breast-feeding increased in duration (Figure 3), and both cow's milk and gluten were introduced later to the babies. The duration of mixed feeding, i.e. when breast-milk is given together with cow's milk and gluten tended to be longer towards the latter part of the observation years (though statistically n.s., Figure 4). However, these associations are hard to relate as the cause or causes of the increased incidence of CD.

TABLE I BIRTH PREVALENCE RATE (BPR) PER 1,000 LIVE BIRTHS.

Year of birth	Total number	BPR	Moving BPR per 3 y.
1970	4	0.62	
1971	5	0.75	
1972	10	1.60	0.98
1973	10	1.68	1.37
1974	4	0.67	1.37
1975	4	0.72	1.09
1976	11	2.10	1.13
1977	10	1.96	1.57
1978	8	1.63	1.90
1979	7	1.38	1.66
1980	5	0.99	1.33
1981	6	1.22	1.20
1982	12	2.35	1.52
1983	12	2.48	2.02
1984	9	1.74	2.18
1985	20	3.75	2.67
1986	15	2.76	2.76
1987	16	2.72	3.07
1988	15	2.44	2.63
Total	183		

Has then the quantity of gluten consumed changed over the time period? The four day records of the dietary intake indicate that this is the case (Table II).
During the eighties the 12 months old infants consumed on an average 50% more gluten compared to the equally old infants 10 years earlier. For 18 months old children the difference was not statistically significant. Why then has the consumption of gluten increased? The studies did not reveal any major change of feeding patterns, but there had been a change of the industrial process in the manufacturing of the

favourite commercial baby foods consumed, i.e. gruels and porridges. The result was on an average a doubling of the gluten contents. This change took place 1982-1983. However, the increase had obviously started before this change occurred, and, in addition, it has continued afterwards. There is thus a cause for further search of factors contributing to the increase.

FIGURE III

DURATION OF BREAST-FEEDING AND AGE AT THE INTRODUCTION OF COW'S MILK AND GLUTEN INTO THE DIETS OF THE CHILDREN WITH CD. MEAN VALUES INDICATED RELATED TO BIRTH YEAR.

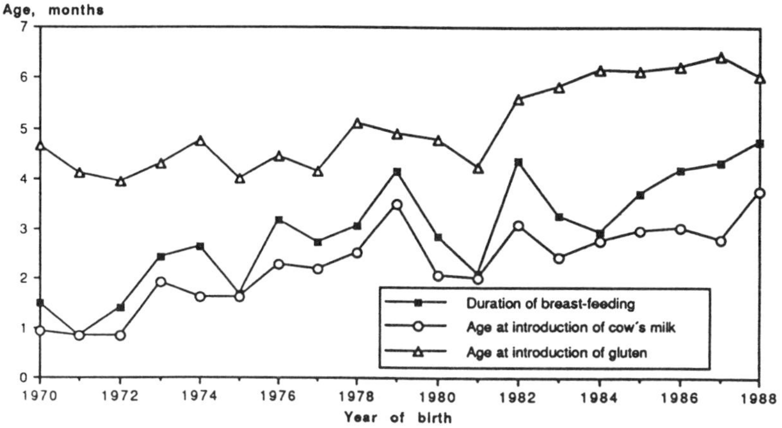

FIGURE IV

DURATION OF BREAST-FEEDING MIXED WITH COW'S MILK AND GLUTEN IN CHILDREN WITH CD. MEAN VALUES RELATED TO BIRTH YEAR.

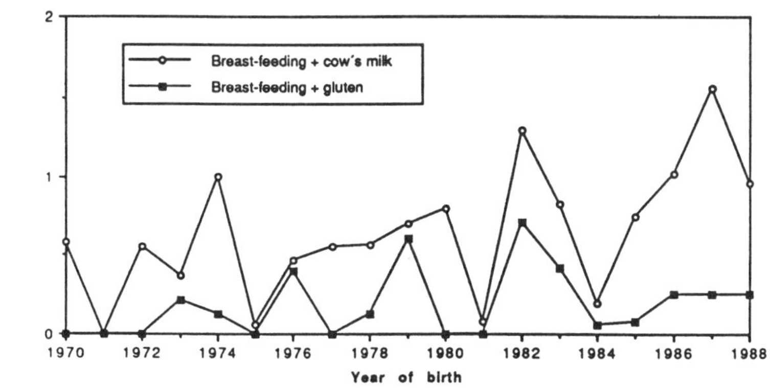

MAY ADENOVIRUS 12 INFECTIONS BE ON THE INCREASE?

Our data with neutralizing tests of antibodies against adenovirus 12 does not support such a hypothesis. We have simply been unable to show any relation between CD and the occurrence of antibodies.

TABLE II PROLAMIN IN GRAM PER DAY, ESTIMATED FROM 4 DAY RECORDS OF DIETARY INTAKE.

Year	Age	Amount	Age	Amount
1978	12 m	1.80	18 m	2.17
1989	12 m	2.72	18 m	2.72
p		0.006		n.s.

n.s. = not significant

MAY DETECTION BIAS EXPLAIN THE INCREASE?

The widespread use of gliadin antibodies determinations among pediatricians and practitioners may certainly lead to increased diagnostic activities, and we do perform an increasing number of small intestinal biopsies. In Sweden 98% of all children are regularly examined and weighed at the Child Health Centres, and the values are plotted in a growth chart on which the rate of increase easily can be assessed. Growth deviations might be identified earlier than in many other places. May we also catch a population with more modest clinical forms of CD? We used growth, or more precisely weight attained at the diagnosis, expressed in SD score, as a marker of the clinical condition (Figure 5). To a significant, though small extent the increase might be due to the recruitment of children with slighter clinical manifestations of CD.

Finally, throughout the study period the children have had the same frequencies of the HLA antigens A1, B8, DR3, DR5 and DR7, all well known to be associated with CD. All children were positive for DRw52, 92% for DR3, 66% for B8 and 57% for A1. The HLA typing has not discovered any finding in favor of the hypothesis that the increased consumption of gluten might induce CD in children without the established genetic predisposition.

CONCLUSION

In conclusion, we have shown that childhood CD is on the increase in the population. CD is now the most common chronic childhood disease in Sweden. The increased consumption of gluten due to the use of industrial baby foods is thought to be the most important contributing factor. We believe that we may approach the true incidence of the disease in our population; in a study of blood donors in Sweden the frequency was actually the same as we currently find (7). In addition, both a

professional and public awareness about the disease may have added to the increase by investigating children with more modest symptoms and who previously may have been unnoticed. There is thus a detection bias contributing to the increase. We have no data to recommend that the current consumption should be decreased. We believe it is an advantage to get the diagnosis at an early age, to avoid protracted ill health later, including the risks of malignancies (8).
The relation between genetic predisposition, gluten exposition and the acquisition of CD is unclear and the problem whether the genetically predisposed individual may avoid CD by consuming low levels of gluten is still unresolved.

FIGURE V

WEIGHT ATTAINED IN CHILDREN <2 YEARS OF AGE AT THE TIME OF THE FIRST SMALL INTESTINAL BIOPSY.
SD-scores. Each square indicates 1-3 individuals.

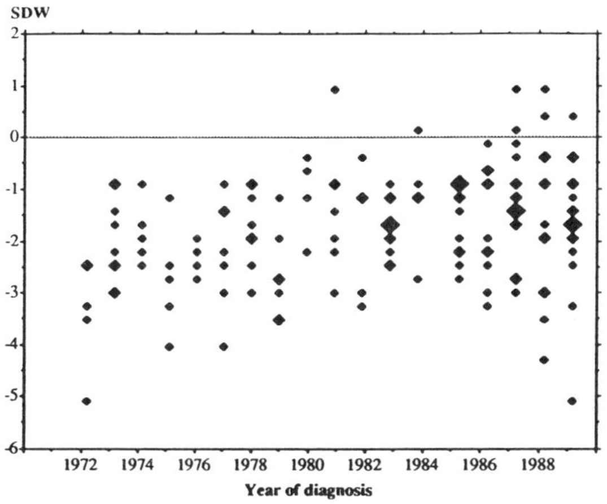

REFERENCES

1 Littlewood JM, Crollick AJ, Richards IDG. Childhood coeliac disease is disappearing. Lancet 1980;ii:1359.
2 Logan RFA, Rifkind EA, Busuttil A, Gilmour HM, Ferguson A. Prevalence and "incidence" of coeliac disease in Edinburgh and Lothian region of Scotland. Gastroenterology 1986;90:334-342.
3 Stevens FM, Egan-Mithcell B, Cryan E, McCarthy CF, McNicholl B. Decreasing incidence of coeliac disease. Arch Dis Child 1987;62:465-468.
4 Mäki M, Kallonen K, Lähdeaho M-L, Visakorpi JK. Changing pattern of childhood coeliac disease in Finland. Acta Paediatr Sand 1988;77:408-412.
5 Greco L, Tozzi AE, Mayer M, Grimaldi M, Silano G, Auricchio S. Unchanging clinical picture of coeliac disease presentation in Campania, Italy. Eur J Pediatr 1989;148:610-613.
6 Kagnoff MF, Austin RK, Hubert JJ, Bernadin JE, Kasarda DD. Possible role for a human adenovirus in the pathogenesis of coeliac disease. J Exp Med 1984;160:1544-1557.
7 Hed J, Lieden G, Ottosson E, Ström M, Walan A, Groth O, Sjögren F, Franzén L. IgA anti-

gliadin antibodies and jejunal mucosal lesions in healthy blood donors. Lancet 1986;ii:215.
8 Holmes GKT, Prio P, Lane MR, Pope P, Allan RN. Malignancy in coeliac disease - effect of a gluten free diet. Gut 1989;30:333-338.

CATCH-UP GROWTH IN 60 CHILDREN WITH COELIAC DISEASE.

G.M. Damen, B. Boersma, J.M. Wit, H.S.A. Heijmans. Dep. Paediatrics, University Utrecht and Groningen, The Netherlands.

Institution of a gluten-free diet in children with coeliac disease (CD) usually results in catch-up growth. However the number of studies on this subject is limited. In a retrospective study among members of the Dutch Coeliac Society 60 CD patients aged 2-20 years were studied. Their diagnosis had been confirmed by means of small bowel biopsies. Height was compared to national standards and expressed as standard deviation scores (SDS). In addition SDS were corrected for parental height in 57 children (95%). In most children (90%) the diagnosis was made between 0.5-3.0 years; 6 children were diagnosed between 5.0-9.0 years. Follow-up ranged between 1.2-10.7 years (average 5.2 years). At the time of diagnosis 20 children (33%) had a SDS below -2.0. All growth data were assessed cross-sectionally with reference to the start of therapy. Generally catch-up growth is complete in 2-3 years. We also studied individual growth curves and formed three groups. Group I, 44 patients (73%), was defined by a positive change in SDS of more than 1.0. Within this group at the time of diagnosis 19 children had a SDS below -2.0 (group Ia), 22 children between -2.0-0.0 (group Ib) and 3 children above 0.0 (group Ic). Group II, 12 patients (20%), was defined by a positive change in SDS of less than 1.0. Group III, 4 patients (7%), was defined by a decrease in SDS. Growth-data of group Ia showed that the average pattern seems to reach a plateau at approximately -1.0 SD after 2 years. The average pattern of group Ib and Ic combined stabilizes around approximately 0.5 SD after 2 years. In group II height catches up very quickly and stabilizes around 0.0 SD in 1-2 years. In group III the growth-pattern of the children seems to be compatible with an absence of stunting before therapy. Of the children diagnosed after the age of 5 years four had a catch-up growth in 1.25-2.25 years, one in 4.5 years and one belonged to group III. Last height SDS measured before the age of 11 and 12 years in girls and boys respectively, were higher than -2.0 (average 0.14) except one child. This study confirms earlier findings that generally in most children with coeliac disease and growth retardation catch-up growth is complete within 2 years, even after an large diagnostic delay.

M. L. Mearin and C. J. J. Mulder (eds.), Coeliac Disease, 115–116.

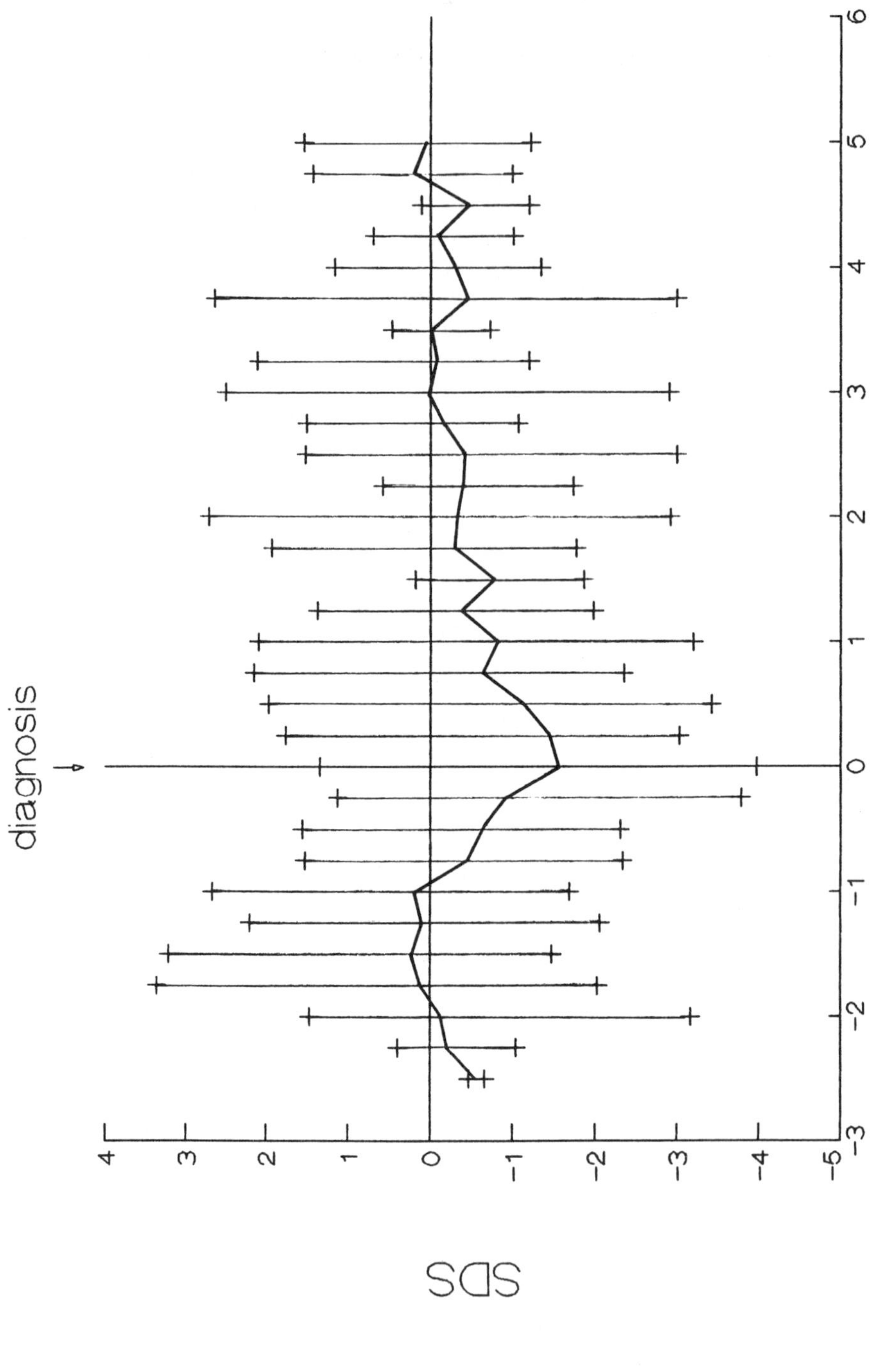

FIGURE

CLINICAL FEATURES OF ADULT COELIAC DISEASE IN ITALY.

G.R. Corazza, M. Frisoni, E.A. Treggiari, R.A. Valentini, C. Filipponi, G. Gasbarrini.
I Medical Pathology, University of Bologna and Department of Internal Medicine and Public Health, University of L'Aquila, Italy.

Over a period of 18 years (1972/1989) we have diagnosed 226 cases of adult coeliac disease (CD), based on biopsy results. The female/male ratio is 2.4 : 1 and the average age in years at the time of diagnosis 36.8 ± 15. The duodenal/jejunal histology of the first biopsy showed subtotal villous atrophy in 209 cases (92%) and partial villous atrophy in the remaining 17 (8%). Diarrhoea and weight loss were the main presenting symptoms in 70% of our patients. Fifteen of our 226 patients died during the survey period and 66% of them had evidence of splenic hypofunction and/or splenic atrophy. Malignancy accounted for 6 deaths.

INTRODUCTION

The first description of the clinical features of adult CD dates back to a century ago (1) and has proved surprisingly up to date until a few years ago. More recent clinical reports, however, have contributed to a change of the classical concepts (2) as, more and more frequently, coeliac patients are described who lack the typical picture of malabsorption (3,4). The aim of this work has been to re-evaluate the clinical features of a large series of adult coeliac patients diagnosed in the last 18 years in an Italian teaching hospital.

MATERIALS AND METHODS

The clinical records of 226 consecutive adult coeliac patients diagnosed in the period 1972-1989 have been reviewed. The diagnosis of CD was accepted if the histology of the intestinal biopsy showed partial or subtotal villous atrophy and such change reverted to normal, or near normal, on a gluten-free diet. An analysis of sex, age at diagnosis, presenting symptoms, associated conditions and mortality has been performed.

RESULTS

One hundred and fifty-nine out of the 226 adult coeliac patients were females with a female/male ratio of 2.4. The mean age at diagnosis was 36.8± 15 years. The frequency distribution of our patients according to sex and age at diagnosis is shown in the figure I.

The duodenal/jejunal histology of the first biopsy showed subtotal villous atrophy in 209 cases (92%) and partial villous atrophy in the remaining 17 (8%); in nine of the latter an associated dermatitis herpetiformis was present. Table I shows the frequency of presenting symptoms in our series, compared to that of six other large series of patients diagnosed by intestinal biopsy. In all these series the most frequent symptoms were diarrhoea and weight loss. 30% of our patients did not present with these symptoms but were diagnosed due to associated diseases, such as dermatitis herpeti-

M. L. Mearin and C. J. J. Mulder (eds.), Coeliac Disease, 117–121.

formis, or to mild blood abnormalities, positive family history, the reduction of Kerckring folds at duodenoscopy (11, 12). A proportion of our patients presented associated diseases (Table II).

The most frequently associated gastrointestinal disorders were bile stones (9 cases), peptic ulcer (9 cases) and pancreatic insufficiency (5 cases); two patients presented macroamylasemia and only one inflammatory bowel disease. The most frequently associated skin disorders were dermatitis herpetiformis (17 cases) and eczema (6 cases); two patients presented pyoderma gangrenosum and one hypertrichosis lanuginosa. The frequent association of CD with atopy has been confirmed in our series, too. Of the 13 patients with associated liver disorders 11 had chronic active hepatitis and two primary biliary cirrhosis.

Among the ten patients with associated thyroid disorders we have found five cases of simple goiter, two of Graves disease, two of Hashimoto thyroiditis and one of follicular carcinoma. Of the seven patients with associated neurological disturbances five had epilepsy and two chorea.

FIGURE I FREQUENCY DISTRIBUTION OF 226 ADULT COELIAC PATIENTS (159 FEMALES AND 67 MALES) ACCORDING TO AGE AT DIAGNOSIS.

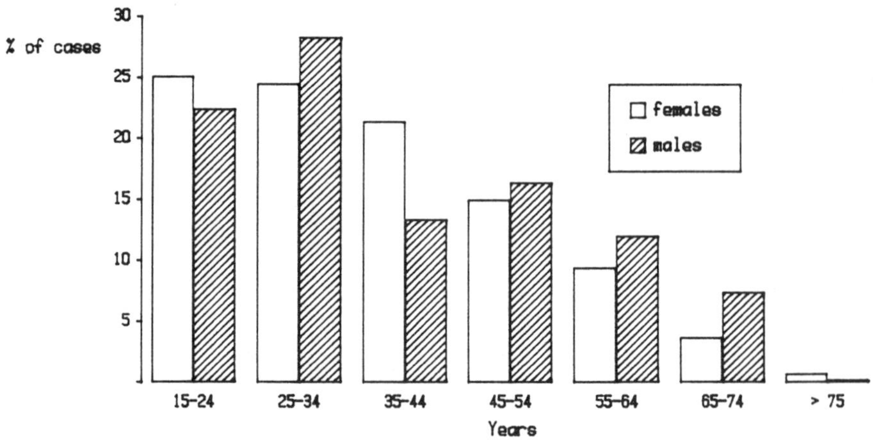

Fifteen of our 226 patients died during the survey period, and the causes of death are listed in Table III. The female/male ratio was 1.1 and the mean age at diagnosis was 52.9±12 years, which was significantly higher ($p<0.01$) than that of the whole series (36.8±15 years). Of these patients 8 out of 12 (66%) -in three of them no data on splenic function were available- had evidence of splenic hypofunction and/or splenic atrophy, but only in patient number 10 death has been confidently related to impaired splenic function (13).

TABLE I FREQUENCY (%) OF PRESENTING SYMPTOMS IN SEVEN DIFFERENT SERIES OF ADULT COELIAC PATIENTS.

Reference	5 (-)	6 (38)	7 (144)	8 (171)	9 (168)	10 (414)	Bologna (226)
Diarrhoea	78	53	73	62	70	80	70
Weight loss	50	47	62	41	62	69	70
Abdominal distension	24	18	70	40	23	-	54
Abdominal pain	-	26	-	43	42	-	50
Constipation	-	-	33	9	-	-	3
Nausea/Vomiting	32	18	32	26	18	-	18
Weakness	-	-	70	61	79	-	73
Bone pain	2	5	-	13	8	-	27
Oedema	16	-	32	5	10	-	27
Muscle cramps /Tetany	-	3	50	-	4	-	20
Menstrual irregularities	-	-	-	30	-	-	23
Aphthous stomatitis	-	-	61	-	28	40	12
Finger clubbing	-	-	-	-	-	-	15
Short stature	-	-	-	19	-	-	6

Figures in brackets indicate the number of cases in each series.

TABLE II ASSOCIATED CONDITIONS IN 226 ADULT COELIAC PATIENTS.

Associated condition	No. of cases	Associated condition	No. of cases
Gastrointestinal disorders	39	Pterygium	4
Skin disorders	37	Renal stones	4
Atopic disorders	15	Vasculitis	4
Liver disorders	13	Psychiatric disorders	3
Thyroid disorders	10	Pericarditis	1
Neurologic disorders	7	Osteogenesis imperfecta	1
Thrombophlebitis	6	IgA deficiency	1
Type I diabetes mellitus	5	Schönlein-Henoch syndrome	1

TABLE III MAIN CLINICAL FEATURES OF 15 ADULT COELIAC PATIENTS WHO DIED DURING THE PERIOD OF SURVEY.

Case	Cause of death	Sex	Diagnosis age	Death age	Spleen state
1.	Intestinal lymphoma	M	49	50	Eusplenic
2.	Intestinal lymphoma	M	56	58	Hyposplenic
3.	Intestinal lymphoma	F	53	54	Not assessed
4.	Intestinal lymphoma	M	70	71	Not assessed
5.	Ulcerative j.ileitis	F	57	61	Not assessed
6.	Ulcerative j.ileitis	F	47	62	Hyposplenic
7.	Liver carcinoma	F	64	64	Eusplenic
8.	Gastric cancer	M	42	44	Eusplenic
9.	Collagenous sprue	M	47	52	Hyposplenic
10.	Lobar pneumonia	F	52	56	Spleen atrophy
11.	Cachexia	F	61	63	Eusplenic
12.	Cachexia	F	50	51	Hyposplenic
13.	Heart failure	M	64	66	Spleen atrophy
14.	Severe hypokalaemia	M	20	27	Hyposplenic
15.	Unknown	F	62	64	Hyposplenic

DISCUSSION

In our 226 consecutive adult coeliac patients the female/male ratio was remarkably high, close to that reported by some authors (3,6), but fairly higher than the overall ratio obtained from 18 previous studies reviewed by Cooke and Holmes (8). As far as age at diagnosis is concerned, the majority of our patients were diagnosed in the third and fourth decades. The lower prevalence of males in our series may explain why we have not found a bimodal distribution of age as previously reported (8). In fact the later peak has been said to be mostly accounted for by males (3) and then, although in our series after the age of 45 the proportion of males was higher than that of females, due to the low absolute number of males the later peak of age incidence was not observed. No remarkable differences in the frequency of presenting symptoms were found between our study and some previous large series of biopsy-proven adult coeliac patients. Differences in the definition of the various symptoms from author to author may partly account for the differences observed. Thirty per cent of our patients did not show the classical features of malabsorption, a proportion lower than that reported in other series (3,4). A good number of our patients had conditions already known to be associated with coeliac disease (14). It is of interest the association with pterygium in four patients and with pyoderma gangrenosum in two others, conditions that to our knowledge have never been related to CD. A recent study has shown that CD brings about an almost twofold increase of overall mortality (15). Our uncontrolled study seems to support that this condition has a generally increased risk of developing cancer (16) and that intestinal lymphoma is the most frequent malignancy (17). It is remarkable that the duration of exposure to gluten in our patients with premature death was longer than that of the whole series, and that

66% of them had splenic hypofunction compared to 32% of all our coeliacs who had splenic function assessed (18). Further studies are needed to clarify whether splenic hypofunction contributes to worsening in some way the natural history of CD or whether it too can be considered as one of the consequences of a longer exposure to gluten.

REFERENCES

1 Gee S. On the coeliac affection. St Bart's Hosp Rep 1888;24:17-20.
2 Vogten AJM, Peña AS. Coeliac disease: one century after Samuel Gee (1988). Neth J Med 1987;31:253-255.
3 Swinson CM, Levi AJ. Is coeliac disease underdiagnosed? Br Med J 1980;281:1258-1260.
4 Logan RFA, Tucker G, Rifkind EA, Heading RC, Ferguson A. Changes in clinical features of coeliac disease in adults in Edinburgh and the Lothians 1960-79. Br Med J 1983;286:95-97.
5 Barry RE, Baker PG, Read AE. The clinical presentation. Clin Gastroenterol 1974;3:55-69.
6 Dissanayake AS, Truelove SC, Whitehead R. Jejunal mucosal recovery in coeliac disease in relation to the degree of adherence to a gluten free diet. Quart J Med 1974;43:161-185.
7 Stevens FM. Celiac disease: clinical manifestations. Pract Gastroenterol 1980;4:10-15.
8 Cooke WT, Holmes GKT. Coeliac disease. Churchill Livingstone, Edinburgh, 1984.
9 Dawson AM, Kumar PJ. Coeliac disease. In: Disorders of the Small Intestine, CC Booth, G Neale (eds). Blackwell, Oxford, 1985,153-178.
10 Biemond I, Peña AS, Groenland F, Mulder CJJ, Tytgat GNJ. Coeliac disease in the Netherlands: demographic data of a patient survey among the members of the Dutch Coeliac Society. Neth J Med 1987;31:263-268.
11 Brocchi E, Corazza GR, Caletti G, Treggiari EA, Barbara L, Gasbarrini G. Endoscopic demonstration of loss of duodenal folds in the diagnosis of celiac disease. N Engl J Med 1989;321:741-744.
12 Corazza GR, Brocchi E, Caletti G, Gasbarrini G. Loss of duodenal folds allows diagnosis of unsuspected coeliac disease. Gut, 1990;31:1080-1081.
13 Corazza GR, Frisoni M, Vaira D, Gasbarrini G. Fatal pneumonia in a patient with coeliac disease and splenic atrophy. Ital J Gastroenterol 1984;16:300-301.
14 Mulder CJJ, Tytgat GNJ. Coeliac disease and related disorders. Neth J Med 1987; 31:286-299.
15 Logan RFA, Rifkind EA, Turner ID, Ferguson A. Mortality in celiac disease. Gastroenterology 1989;97:265-271.
16 Nielsen OH, Jacobsen O, Rask Pedersen E, Norby Rasmussen S, Petri M, Laulund S, Jarnum S. Non-tropical sprue. Malignant diseases and mortality rate. Scand J Gastroenterol 1985;20:13-18.
17 Swinson CM, Slavin G, Coles EC, Booth CC. Coeliac disease and malignancy. Lancet 1983;1:111-115.
18 Corazza GR, Amorosa L, Strocchi A, Zoli G, Mantovani V, Gasbarrini G. Assessment of prevalence, familial occurrence and possible factors inducing splenic hypofunction in adult coeliac disease in Italy. Gut 1989;30:1452-1453.

ASSOCIATED DISEASES IN CHILDREN WITH COELIAC DISEASE.

Isabel Polanco, G. Prieto, Rosa Lama, Sira Carrasco, Rosa Codoceo, J. Larrauri.
Department of Paediatrics. Gastroenterology Unit. Hospital Infantil "La Paz", Facultad de Medicina. Universidad Autónoma. Madrid, Spain.

Coeliac disease (CD) in adults has been reported in association with a variety of conditions, some of them autoallergic, and others with an unspecified aetiology. However no systematic prevalence data have been published in large series of coeliac children.
The aim of this study was to estimate the frequency and nature of associated diseases in our series of coeliac patients and to study the possible influence of the HLA-DR phenotypes in this population. The clinical history of 440 coeliac patients (269 females and 171 males) diagnosed according to the ESPGAN criteria were analized. In 44 of them (18 males an 26 females) another diagnosis was established. The overall incidence of associated diseases was 10%. The following entities were found: Isolated IgA deficiency (12 cases), asthma (6), dermatitis herpetiformis (6), diabetes mellitus type I (5), chronic active hepatitis (4), psoriasis (4), congenital heart disease (3), vitiligo (2), cystic fybrosis (1), fibrosing alveolitis (1). There were no significant differences in sex distribution. In four patients the clinical manifestations of the associated disease began together with the gluten challenge. The results suggest an influence of the HLA-DR phenotypes in the frequence of the associated disease. The gluten challenge could be contraindicated in those coeliac patients with an associated severe disease. Additional prevalence-data on associated diseases in childhood CD are needed.

INTRODUCTION

The pathogenesis of CD is still unknown. However, the interaction among genetic, immunological and environmental factors seems to play a role in the expression of CD (1-16). Many disorders have been reported in association with CD in adults (17-19), but prevalence data on associated diseases in large series of coeliac children have not been published.
The occurence of CD in association with other disorders is possibly underestimated, because CD may be asymptomatic (20-24) and because the clinical picture of a coeliac patient may be attributed to the associated disease alone. In active CD numerous immunological alterations, including a number of autoimmune diseases, have been found (19,25-32). Isolated case reports of non-immunological disorders associated with CD have been published too (32-35). In CD, the presence of certain HLA-DR phenotypes seems to exert some influence on the clinical course. For example, monosymptomatic forms of CD are more frequent among male coeliac children with phenotypes HLA-DR3/ other HLA-DR and HLA- DR7/other HLA-DR than among those with HLA-DR3/ DR7 (9,10,21). In our experience coeliac patients who are DR3/DR3 show a more rapid clinical, functional and histological relapse, after gluten challenge (10,23). Prolonged breast feeding appears to cause a delay on the onset of symptoms in those patients having phenotypes DR3/DR3,

M. L. Mearin and C. J. J. Mulder (eds.), Coeliac Disease, 123–129.

DR3/DR7 and DR7/ DR5 (13). It has been shown too that the HLA-DR status of the patients exerts some influence on their antigliadin antibodies serum levels (29).

AIM: The aim of this study was to estimate the frequency and nature of the associated diseases in our series of coeliac children and to study the possible influence of their HLA-DR phenotypes on the prevalence of the associated conditions.

PATIENTS AND METHODS: In the last 20 years (1967-1987) we have diagnosed and followed 440 cases of well established CD. In all the cases the diagnosis of CD has been made according to the ESPGAN criteria (i.e., small bowel villous atrophy at presentation, normal mucosa after withdrawal of gluten from the diet, and relapse of mucosal abnormalities after reintroduction of gluten) (36,37). Small bowel biopsies were obtained from beyond the ligament of Treitz using a Watson Paediatric capsule. All the histological sections were evaluated at the Department of Histopathology of the University Hospital "La Paz" in Madrid, whose help is herewith acknowledged.

RESULTS: Of the 440 coeliac children (269 girls, 171 boys), 44 of them (26 girls, 18 boys) were found to have an associated disorder (Table I).

TABLE I ASSOCIATED DISORDERS IN COELIAC CHILDREN (ESPGAN CRITERIA)

Selective IgA deficiency	12
Bronchial asthma	6
Dermatitis herpetiformis	6
Diabetes mellitus	5
Chronic active hepatitis	4
Psoriasis	4
Cardiovascular disease	3
Vitiligo	2
Cystic fibrosis	1
Fibrosing alveolitis	1
TOTAL	44 (= 10%)

TABLE II ASSOCIATED DISORDERS IN CHILDREN WITH A POSSIBLE CD

Diabetes mellitus	4
Dermatitis herpetiformis	3
Down's syndrome	3
Renal tubular defects	2
Alpha-1-AT deficiency	1
Schönlein-Henoch purpura	1

The overall incidence of associated diseases is 10%, but it may be higher, if we consider fourteen other patients with suspected CD who have not been challenged with gluten yet (Tabel II).

The commonest association found was isolated IgA deficiency. None of the six patients with dermatitis herpetiformis presented gastrointestinal symptoms, although four of them had steatorrhoea, high levels of antireticulin antibodies (ARA) and a flat small intestine mucosa. The other two patients had only a partial villous atrophy, but they showed a flat mucosa after gluten challenge. Other skin disorders, like psoriasis and vitiligo were also found, as described in adult patients. One case of cystic fibrosis and three cases of congenital heart diseases have been also encountered. A pair of monozygotic twins concordant for CD (5) developed juvenile diabetes mellitus simultaneously, and later on, simultaneously too, a persistent leukopenia. In all four coeliac children with chronic active hepatitis liver biopsy showed peacemeal necrosis in the portal tracts. Fibrosing alveolitis in a girl with CD was recognized. The histological features at lung biopsy were thickening of alveolar walls and presence of large mononuclear cells in the alveolar spaces.
Tables III and IV show the distribution of the HLA-DR phenotypes in the representative sample of Spanish coeliac children and controls, and the distribution of the HLA-DR phenotypes of the CD patients with and without associated disorders.

TABLE III HLA-DR PHENOTYPES DISTRIBUTION IN COELIAC PATIENTS AND CONTROLS

HLA-DR phenotypes	Patients (n=163) (+)	(%)	Controls (n=76) (+)	(%)	Significance p	R.R.**
DR3/und.	20	12.3	0	0.0	4.10-2	21.8
DR3/DR5	12	7.4	4	5.2	n.s.	1.4
DR3/DR7	62	38.0	2	2.6	2.10-7	11.5
DR3/other	22	13.4	7	9.2	n.s.	1.5
DR5/und.	0	0.0	1	1.3	n.s.	0.2
DR5/DR7	30	18.4	4	5.6	n.s.	3.7
DR5/other	5	3.1	13	17.1	4.10-3	0.2
DR7/und.	2	1.2	4	5.3	n.s.	0.2
DR7/other	6	3.7	19	25.0	2.10-5	0.1
Other/other	4	2.4	22	28.9	4.10-8	0.1

und = HLA not determined; ** = relative risk for CD

There was a HLA-DR3/DR7 phenotype predominance in the associated disease group ($p<0.025$). We found two coeliac siblings (girl and boy) who shared only one HLA-DR antigen (DR3). The girl was DR3/DR7 and had dermatitis herpetiformis. Diabetes mellitus type I was recently diagnosed in her brother (DR3/DR4).

TABLE IV HLA-DR PHENOTYPES DISTRIBUTION IN PATIENTS WITH AND WITHOUT ASSOCIATED DISEASES

HLA-DR phenotypes	With associated diseases (n=44)	Without associated diseases (n=315)
DR3/undetermined	7 %	12 %
DR3/DR5	4.5 %	7 %
DR3/DR7	63.8 % **	38 %
DR3/other *	18 %	13 %
DR5/DR7	7 %	19 %
DR5/other *	-	3 %
DR7/undetermined	-	1.5 %
DR7/other *	-	3.5 %
Other/other *	-	3 %

* Other = antigen differing from DR3, DR5 or DR7; ** $p < 0.025$

DISCUSSION

The association between CD and other autoimmune diseases is well known and supports the existence of an altered immunological respons in coeliac patients.
Knowledge of the frequency and characteristics of the associated entities, can improve the understanding of the pathogenesis of CD. These associations have been possibly underestimated since CD can be asymptomatic and because it is difficult to recognize a patient suffering from two different diseases at the same time. For years dermatitis herpetiformis (DH) has been considered an exclusively dermatological disorder, however we come to recognize it as CD of the skin. Patients with DH rarely consult the gastroenterologist because of gastro-intestinal symptoms. The presence of villous damage in almost all cases of DH and its evident improvement together with the improvement of the cutaneous lesions after a gluten free diet, makes clear its close relationship with CD. The association between CD and a selective IgA deficiency is even closer, considering the relative low frequency of both entities.
In infancy and young adults the association between CD and diabetes mellitus type I is relatively frequent. In adult coeliac patients, other less common associations have been described: fibrosing alveolitis, Sjögren's syndrome, inflammatory bowel disease, autoimmune thyroiditis, rheumatoid arthritis, primary bilairy cirrhosis, etc. (19). Fibrosing alveolitis in infancy and childhood has been reported as a rare condition (38). However, we report the first well documented case in association with CD in childhood.
Cystic fibrosis (39-44) and cardiovascular diseases (19) have been also encountered in association with CD. It is a general opinion that these conditions occur together just by chance. In any case, it seems important to consider the existence of eventually associated diseases when the clinical course is poorly explained by CD alone (17,19,21).

In 4 of our patients (two diabetes mellitus, one cystic fibrosis and the exceptional case of fibrosing alveolitis) the associated disease appeared during gluten challenge. Because of this, we suggest not to challenge these patients.
The relationship between the HLA status of the CD patients and the occurrence or absence of associated diseases in our series have been shown in Table IV. We found an increased number of heterozygotes DR3/DR7 and a decreased number of homozygotes DR7/DR7 in comparision with the controls ($p<0.025$). Although this series is large it is possible that the patients studied do not represent the whole coeliac population. It is possible that patients with phenotype DR7/DR7 may express their symptoms in a "milder way" so that they never undergo intestinal biopsy (9,21,23). It is possible too that some DR3/DR3 patients with an immunological associated disease might be treated because of the immunological disorder and never be diagnosed as having CD.
In our series we have found an incidence of at least 10 per 100 of associated disorders including autoimmune conditions. The present results suggest some influence of the HLA system on the frequency of associated disease. Although we still believe that the histological relapse after gluten challenge is necessary to confirm CD, the challenge with gluten may be contraindicated in CD children with another autoimmune disease or in those with a chronic severe illness.

REFERENCES

1 Dicke WK, Weijers HA, van de Kamer JH. Coeliac disease II. The presence in wheat of a factor having a deleterious effect in cases of coeliac disease. Acta Paediatr 1953; 42:34-42.
2 Stokes PL, Asquith P, Holmes GKT, MacKintosch P, Cooke WT. Histocompatibility antigens associated with adult coeliac disease. Lancet 1972; 11:162-4.
3 Falchuck ZM, Rogentine GN, Strober W. Predominance of histocompatibility antigen HLA-8 in patients with glutensensitive enteropathy. J Clin Invest 1972; 51:1602-5.
4 Keuning JJ, Peña AS, van Leeuwen A, van Hooff JP, van Rood JJ. HLA-DW3 associated with coeliac disease. Lancet 1976; 1:506-7.
5 Polanco I, Biemond I, van Leeuwen A, Schreuder I, Meera Khan P, Guerrero I, D'Amaro I, Vazquez C, van Rood JJ, Peña AS. Gluten sensitive enteropathy in Spain: Genetic and environmental factors. In: RB McConnelled The genetics of coeliac disease. Liverpool. MTP Press 1981; pp:211-34.
6 Mearin ML, Biemond I, Peña AS, Polanco I, Vazquez C, Schreuder I, de Vries RRP, van Rood JJ. HLA-DR phenotypes in Spanish coeliac children: their contribution to the understanding of the genetics of the disease. Gut 1983; 24:532-7.
7 Toso R, Vismara D, Taginaki N, Ferrara GB, Cicimarra F, Baffolano W, Follo D, Auricchio S. Evidence that coeliac disease is primarily associated with a DC locus allelic specificity. Clin Immunol Inmunopathol 1983; 28:395-404.
8 Tosi R, Tanigaki N, Polanco I. DeMarchi M, Woodrow JC, Hetzel PA. A radioimmunoassay typing study of non-DQw2-associated coeliac disease. Clin Immunol Inmunopathol 1986; 39:168-72.
9 DeMarchi M, Carbonara A, Ansaldi N, Santini B, Barbera C, Borelli I, Rossino P, Rendine S. HLA-DR3 and DR7 in coeliac disease: inmunogenetic and clinical aspects. Gut 1983; 24: 706-12.
10 Polanco I. Aspectos genéticos y ambientales de la enfermedad celiaca. Doctoral thesis. 1980. University of Madrid, Spain.
11 Polanco I, Vazquez C, Guerrero J, Carrasco S, Prieto G, Peña AS. Concordance and disconcordance of coeliac disease in monozygotic twins. Acta Paediatr Belg 1979; 32:152-3.
12 Polanco I, Vazquez C. The influence of breast feeding in coeliac disease. Paediatr Res 1981; 15:1193A.

13 Polanco I, Vazquez C, Prieto G, Carrasco S, Mearin ML, Peña AS. Coeliac disease: influence of breast feeding and HLA-DR phenotypes on the age of onset of symptoms. Paediatr Res 1982; 16:1044A.
14 Auricchio S, Follo D, de Ritis G, Giunta A, Marzorati D. Workin hypothesis: Does breast feeding protect against the development of clinical symptoms of coeliac disease in children? J Pediatr Gastroenterol Nutr 1983; 2:428-33.
15 Kagnoff MF, Austin RK, Mubert JJ, Bernardin JE, Kasarda DD. Possible role for a human adenovirus in the pathogenesis of coeliac disease. J Exp Med 1984; 160:1544-57.
16 Polanco I, Mearin ML, Larrauri J, Biemond I, Wipkink-Bakker A, Peña AS. Effect of gluten supplementation in health siblings of children with coeliac disease. Gastroenterology 1987; 92:678-81.
17 Scott BB, Losowsky MS. Coeliac disease: a cause of various associated diseases. Lancet 1975; ii:956-7.
18 Mulder CJJ, Giard RWM, Peña AS, Weterman IT. Coeliac disease and ulcerative colitis: a diagnostic pitfall. Nether J med 1983; 26:80-3.
19 Cooke WT, Holmes GR. Coeliac disease. Edinburgh, Churchill Living-stone, 1984; pp:225-46.
20 Congdon P, Mason MK, Smith S. Small intestinal bowel mucosa in asymptomatic children with coeliac disease. Am J Dis Child 1981; 135:118-21.
21 Polanco I. Enfermedad celiaca. In: C Chantar, J Rodés, eds. Actualidades en gastroenterologia. Barcelona. Prous 1986; pp:1-37.
22 Ansaldi N, Santini B, Barbera C, Dell'Olio D, Borelli I, DeMarchi M, Richardi P. HLA and coeliac disease: correlation with its clinical and histological aspects. Ped Med Chir 1979; 1:381-4.
23 Polanco I: Factores genéticos Y ambientales en la enfermedad celiaca. In: M Diaz Rubio, ed. Avances en gastroenterologia. Madrid. Jarpyo Ed. SA. 1985; pp:133-46.
24 Auricchio S, Massacca G, Tosi R, Visakorpi J, Mäki M, Polanco I. Coeliac disease as familial condition: Identification of asymptomatic coeliac patients within family groups. Gastroenterology International 1988; 1:25-31.
25 Cooper BT, Holmes GKT, Cooke WT. Coeliac disease and immunological disorders. Br Med J 1978; 1:537-9.
26 Savilhati E, Perkkio M, Kalimo L, Vainio E, Renala T. IgA antigliadin antibodies: a marker of mucosal damage in childhood coeliac disease. Lancet 1983; i:320-2.
27 Unsworth DJ, Walker-Smith JA, Holborow EJ. Gliadin and reticulin antibodies in childhood coeliac disease. Lancet 1983; i:874-6.
28 Ribes-Koninckx C, Giliams JP, Polanco I, Peña AS. IgA antigliadin antibodies in coeliac and inflammatory bowel disease. J Pediatr Gastroenterol Nutr 1984; 3:676-82.
29 Mearin ML, Ribes-Koninckx C, Biemond I, Polanco I, Peña AS. Influence of genetic factors on the serum levels of antigliadin antibodies in coeliac disease. J Pediatr Gastroenterol Nutr 1984; 3:373-77.
30 Strober W. Gluten-sensitive enteropathy. An abnormal immunologic response of the gastrointestinal tract to a dietary immunity for the clinician. New York. Grune and Stratton, Inc. 1985; pp:75-112.
31 Walker-Smith JA, Andrews J. Alpha-1 antitrypsin, autism and coeliac disease. Lancet 1972; ii:883-4.
32 Greenwold AJ, Johnson DS, Oskvig RM. Alpha-1 antitrypsin deficiency emphysema, cirrhosis and intestinal mucosal atrophy. JAMA 1975; 231:273-6.
33 Bentley D. A case of Down's syndrome complicated by retinoblastoma and coeliac disease. Pediatrics 1975; 56:131-3.
34 Massa G, Casaer P, Eggermont E. Gluten enteropathy and Charcot-Marie-Tooth disease: an unusual association. Tijdschrift voor Gastroenterologie 1989; 22:151-6.
35 Mulder CJJ, Tytgat GNJ. Coeliac disease and related disorders. Nether J Med 1987; 31:286-99.
36 Meeuwise GW. Diagnostic criteria in coeliac disease. Acta Paediatr Scand 1970; 59:461-3.
37 McNeish AS, Harms HK, Rey J, Shmerling DH, Visakorpi JK, Walker-Smith JA. The diagnosis of coeliac disease. Arch Dis Child 1979; 54:783-6.
38 Hewitt CJ, Huel D, Keeling JW. Fibrosing alveolitis in infancy and childhood. Arch Dis Child

1977; 52:22-37.
39 Hide DW, Burman D. An infant with both cystic fibrosis and coeliac disease. Arch Dis Child 1969; 44:533-5.
40 Taylor B, Sokol G. Cystic fibrosis and coeliac disease: report of two cases. Arch Dis Child 1973; 48:692-6.
41 Goodchild MC, Nelson R, Anderson CM. Cystic fibrosis and coeliac disease: co-existent in two children. Arch Dis Child 1973; 48:684-91.
42 Franklin JL, Asquith P, Rosenberg H. The occurence of cystic fibrosis and coeliac sprue within a single sibship. Am J Dig Dis 1974; 19:149-55.
43 Katz AJ, Falchuk M, Shwachman H: The coexistence of cystic fibrosis and coeliac disease. Pediatrics 1976; 57:715-21.
44 Wauters EAK, van de Kamer JH. Excretion of pyrrolidonyl peptides and aminoacid conjugates in a patient with coeliac disease and cystic fibrosis. In: B McNicholl, CF McCarthy, PF Fotrell, eds. Perspectives in coeliac disease. Lancaster. MTP Press 1977; pp:473-77.

COELIAC DISEASE AND AUTOIMMUNE ENTEROPATHY.

J.A. Walker-Smith, Academic Department of Paediatric Gastroenterology, Queen Elizabeth Hospital for Children Hackney Road, London E2 8PS, UK.

Autoimmune enteropathy is a syndrome which typically presents in early childhood, very similar to coeliac disease, with chronic diarrhoea and failure to thrive. It is associated with a severe small intestinal enteropathy. There is no clinical or histological response to a gluten-free diet or other dietary exclusion. There is evidence of predisposition to autoimmune disease either by the presence of circulating gut and other autoantibodies and/or associated autoimune disease. There is usually no immuno-deficiency. The small intestinal mucosal lesion at time of presentation may be indistinguishable morphologically, on occasion, from untreated coeliac disease (hyperplastic villous atrophy). Furthermore there may be high circulating levels of anti-gliadin antibody. However intraepithelial lymphocyte counts are usually not increased and there was no increased expression of the gamma/delta receptor on intraepithelial lymphocytes in the small intestinal mucosa in three children with autoimmune enteropathy. Study of the intraepithelial lymphocyte count is likely to be a valuable observation to permit differentiation of the two disorders at time of presentations. This disorder needs to be distinguished from a coeliac crisis. The severity of the small intestinal mucosal damage bears no relationship to the presence of the level of circulating gut autoantibodies. Whilst the detection of such antibodies is of diagnostic usefulness, T-cell activation of lymphocytes in the small intestinal mucosa is likely to be more central to pathogenesis of autoimmune enteropathy. Cyclosporin has been effective therapy in three children.

INTRODUCTION

For some time it has been known that there are autoimmune associations of coeliac disease (CD). The first is the well known association of untreated CD with circulating antireticulin antibodies (1,2). Although the precise specificity of R1 anti-reticulin antibody remains unclear (3). General autoantibody screening in CD has also shown that the incidence of antinuclear, antiparietal cell, anti-thyroid and other autoantibodies are increased both in adults and in children (4,5). These were tissue reactive autoantibodies detected by indirect immunofluorescence on frozen sections.

While the R1 anti-reticulin antibody disappears on a gluten-free diet, the other autoantibodies persist. Thus the presence of anti-reticulin antibody appears to reflect gluten exposure in coeliac patients. Whereas the presence of other autoantibodies may reflect an underlying defect of immunoregulation, in a few patients. There have also been several reports of an association between CD and other diseases regarded as autoimmune in origin. These include type I diabetes, thyroiditis and Sjogrens disease (6,7). There is at present however nothing to indicate that the enteropathy of CD per se arises via an autoimmune mechanism.

In 1982, an eighteen month old boy was reported (8) who presented with chronic diarrhoea and failure to thrive, a flat small intestinal mucosa, high circulating titre of IgA antibodies to gliadin and reticulin, suggesting the diagnosis of CD. He failed to

M. L. Mearin and C. J. J. Mulder (eds.), Coeliac Disease, 131–136.

respond to a gluten-free diet and required intravenous alimentation. Subsequently, he was found to have a circulating IgA autoantibody reactive with rat and human gut epithelium. It appeared after initial presentation. He also had evidence of other circulating autoantibodies, including pancreatic islet cell antibody. There was a family history of a sibling dying with flat mucosa and diabetes mellitus. Then at the ESPGAN meeting in Graz, a further 6 similar cases were presented from a number of countries (9). The concept was put forward that autoimmunity plays an important role in the pathogenesis of protacted diarrhoea in some infants and that gut autoantibodies may prove a useful marker of disease.

DIAGNOSTIC CRITERIA

From these observations came the concept of autoimmune enteropathy (5,10). A literature review in 1985 revealed a total of 5 similar published cases. The diagnosis of autoimmune enteropathy had been based upon four criteria (5):

- Presentation with protracted diarrhoea and severe enteropathy
- No response of the disease process to exclusion diet or total parenteral nutrition
- Evidence of predisposition to autoimmune disease.
  Presence of circulatory autoantibodies and or associated autoimmune disease.
- No severe immunodeficiency.

Another case, described by McCarthy (11), who had an unresponsive small intestinal enteropathy associated with an autoantibody to gut epithelium was excluded as the patient had absent serum IgA. Immunodeficiency was believed by the authors to be the predisposing factor. More recently, Catassi (12), have described a child with persistent enteropathy and circulating enterocyte autoantibodies and type I diabetes in a boy with common variable hypogammaglobulinaemia. However it is uncertain whether or not immunodeficiency is associated with autoimmune enteropathy. In the child reported by Catassi it was several years after the diagnosis of hypogammaglobulinaemia was made that he presented with the features of autoimmune enteropathy. It is likely that both the cases described by McCarthy and Catassi did have autoimmune enteropathy. Whether immunodeficiency was coincidental remains unknown at present. In 1986, the largest series to date of children with this disorder were described (13) 14 out of 25 children with chronic diarrhoea and failure to thrive of unknown origin were found to have circulating autoantibodies to enterocytes, none had severe immunodeficiency. All except one had a small intestinal enteropathy on biopsy. This ranged from a flat mucosa to patchy partial villous atrophy. Thirteen had other circulating autoantibodies. Six had evidence of other "autoimmune disease" e.g. diabetes mellitus, rheumatoid arthritis and renal disease.

In general the original diagnostic criteria as proposed in 1985 appear to remain a valid basis for the recognition of this syndrome, although the presence of immunodeficiency should not exclude the diagnosis. However the true nature of autoimmune enteropathy remains elusive and the importance of circulating gut autoantibodies for pathogenesis remains uncertain as the presence of the circulating autoantibody bears no direct relationship to the severity of the small intestinal mucosal lesion (14). Furthermore, its absence does not exclude autoimmune enteropathy as cases have been described where the antibody has not been present at the beginning of the illness. One remarkable child reported by Unsworth-Walker-Smith (5) in 1985, as enteropathy associated with microscopic colitis, developed gut autoantibody years later.

The key experiment to demonstrate that these gut autoantibodies are cytotoxic in small intestinal organ culture system has not yet been done. The increased intensity of the staining of gut epithelial antibodies towards the end of the life of in a child who died has suggested that the autoantibodies may be the effect rather than the cause of widespread organ damage (15). Auto-reactive T cells may play a major role in aetiology as activated T cells are found in this disorder. Indeed in 1983 (9) a hypothesis was put forward that children with autoimmune enteropathy were genetically predisposed to this disorder and that an infectious agent was often a triggering agent. Then related to a defect of immunoregulation, autoantibodies and autoreactive T cells appeared leading to a variety of autoimmune diseases. Although it is likely that autoreactive T cells play a more important role in pathogenesis, nevertheless the presence of a circulating gut autoantibody remains an useful diagnostic marker comparable to the diagnostic value of gliadin antibody in coeliac disease. In a child with an enteropathy unresponsive to dietary elimination the finding of this antibody permits a firm diagnosis of autoimmune enteropathy to be made.

DEFINITION

An autoimmune enteropathy may be defined as a disorder of the small intestinal mucosa where persistent small intestinal mucosal damage occurs as a result of autoimmune mechanisms. The disease may be confined to the small intestine or it may be part of a multisystemic disease process.

SMALL INTESTINAL LESION

It is possible to differentiate the histological lesion of autoimmune enteropathy from untreated CD by morphometric and monoclonal antibody analysis. The mucosa may be completely flat as in untreated CD with the features of hyperplastic villous atrophy. More usually the lesion is less severe and patchy in distribution. The number of intraepithelial lymphocytes are usually not increased as they are in active CD. In fact, gamma-delta expression by these lymphocytes is very low and discriminates these cases from CD (Figure 1) (Spencer 1990 in preparation).

CLINICAL FEATURES

Autoimmune enteropathy classically presents in early infancy but has been reported up to the teenage years although it has not yet been observed to present in adult life. In infancy autoimmune enteropathy may present with the classical features of CD i.e. chronic diarrhoea and failure to thrive, flat small intestinal mucosa, circulating gliadin and reticulin antibodies, but the children do not respond to a gluten-free diet (5).

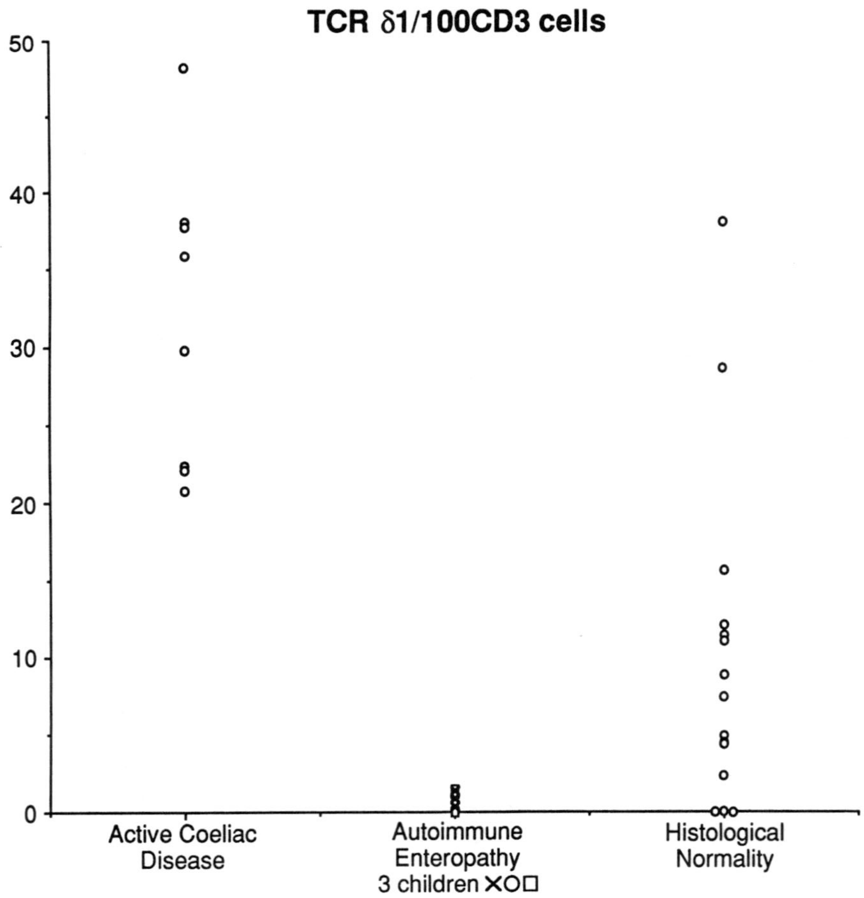

FIGURE I EXPRESSION DELTA-ONE BY T-CELL RECEPTOR FOR 100 INTRAEPITHELIAL LYMPHOCYTES EXPRESSING CD3

Typically there is other organ involvement with diabetes mellitus, interstitial nephropathy, rheumatoid arthritis and hypothyroidism as disease associations. Severe renal involvement is a bad prognostic sign. Circulating thyroid, pancreatic islet cell and renal autoantibodies are common. When low titre gut autoantibodies levels are present and the pathology is confined to the gut, the prognosis is better and spontaneous clinical recovery is possible. Low titre antibody levels may also be found transiently in other enteropathies e.g. cow's milk sensitive enteropathy (13). Indeed it is possible that low titres are a non-specific marker of persistent small intestinal enteropathy, although they have never been found in untreated CD.

MANAGEMENT

Treatment is often unsatisfactory, usually requiring intravenous alimentation, oral steroids and more recently cyclosporin therapy. However in some cases all treatment fails and death is the outcome (13,15). Cyclosporin A has recently been favoured for treatment as cyclosporin A is known to inhibit some effects of T-cell activation. This has been clearly shown in a foetal organ culture test system (16). As T-cell activation may be central to the pathogenesis of this syndrome, cyclosporin A therapy forms a rational basis for management. It is recommended that an initial dose of 100mg/m2/day is given with close monitoring of 10 hour post dose circulating level. A level of 50 ng/ml cyclosporin is recommended. Higher doses are often required to achieve this level because of malabsorption. Using such a regime in two children there was evidence of improved small intestinal structure and function with acceleration of linear growth (17). How long such therapy is required at present remains quite unknown.

Prior to the use of cyclosporin, the mortality from this disease was high with several fatal cases reported in the literature (15,18). Some children are steroid responsive and remain well on a low steroid dosage, others are completely unresponsive to steroids. Spontaneous recovery has been reported (19). Better prognosis is associated with low gut autoantibody titres and localization of pathology to the small intestine. This strange variability in clinical severity is but one of the many mysteries of this strange disorder of childhood which can mimic CD in its presentation.

REFERENCES

1 Brown IL, Ferguson A, Carswell F, Horne CHW, MacSween RNM. Autoantibody in children with coeliac disease. Clin Eur Immunol 1973;13:373.

2 Unsworth DJ, Walker-Smith JA, Holborrow EJ. Gliadin and reticulin antibodies in childhood coeliac disease. Lancet 1983;1:874-875.

3 Unsworth DJ, Scott DL, Walton KW, Walker-Smith JA, Holborrow EJ. Failure of R1 type anti-reticulin antibody to react with fibronectin collagen type III or the non-collagenous reticulin component (NCRC). Clin Exp Imm 1984;57:609-613.

4 Seah PP, Fry L, Hoffbrand AV, Holborrow EJ. Tissue antibodies in dermatitis herpetiformis and adult coeliac disease. Lancet 1971;1:834.

5 Unsworth DJ, Walker-Smith JA.Autoimmunity in diarrhoeal disease. J Pediatr Gastroenterol Nutr 1985;4:375-380.

6 Ferguson A,McNeish AS. Coeliac Disease. Scot M J 1970;15:118.

7 Pittman EF, Holud DA. Sjogren's Syndrome and adult coeliac disease. Gastroenterology 1965;48:869.

8 Walker-Smith JA, Unsworth DJ, Hutchins P, Phillips AD, Holborrow EJ. Autoantibodies against gut epithelium in a child with small intestinal enteropathy. Lancet 1982;1:566-567.
9 Unsworth DJ, Walker-Smith JA, Holborrow EJ, Savage MO, Balder AH, Brown H, Harms HK and Savilhati E. Autoimmunity and protracted diarrhoea - A new entity. Paediatric Research 1983;31:425.
10 Unsworth DJ, Hutchins P, Mitchell J, Phillips SAD, Hindocha P, Holborrow J, Walker-Smith JA. Flat small intestinal mucosa and autoantibodies against the gut epithelium. J Pediatr Gastroenterol Nutr 1982;1:503-513.
11 McCarthy DM, Katz SI, Gazze L, Waldmann TA, Nelson DL, Strober W. Selective IgA deficiency associated with total villous atrophy of the small intestine and an organ-specific anti-epithelial cel antibody. J Immunol 1978;120:932-938.
12 Catassi C, Mirakian R, Natalini G, Sbarbati A, Cinti S, Coppa GV, Giorgi PL. Unresponsive enteropathy associated with circulating enterocyte autoantibodies in a boy with common variable hypogammaglobulinaemia and type I diabetes. J Pediatr Gastroenterol Nutr 1988;7:608-613.
13 Mirakian R, Richardson A, Milla PJ, Walker-Smith JA, Unsworth J, Savage MO, Bottezzo GF. Protracted diarrhoea of infancy. Evidence in support of an autoimmune variant. Br Med J 1986;293:1132-1136.
14 Phillips AD, Walker-Smith JA. Proximal small intestinal mucosal morphology in relation to gut epithelial autoantibodies in children with "autoimmune enteropathy". 1st Joint Meeting BSPG and Italian Society of Paediatric Gastroenterology, Parma 1989.
15 Mitton SG, Mirakian R, Larcher VF, Dillon MJ, Walker-Smith JA. Enteropathy and renal involvement in an infant with evidence of widespread autoimmune disturbance. J Pediatr Gastroentol Nutr 1989;8:397-400.
16 MacDonald TT, Spencer J. Evidence that activated mucosal T-cells play a role in the pathogenesis of enteropathy in human small intestine. J Exp Med 1988; 167:1341-1349.
17 Sanderson IR, Walker-Smith JA, Phillips AD. Response of autoimmune associated enteropathy to cyclosporine therapy. 1990. Submitted for publication.
18 Savilhati E, Peikonen P, Holmberg C, Perkkio M, Unsworth J. Fatal unresponsive villous atrophy of the jejunum, connective tissue disease and diabetes in a girl with intestinal epithealial cell antibody. Acta Paediatr Scand 1985;4:187-195.
19 Savage MO, Mirakian R, Wozniak ER, Jenkins HR, Malone M, Phillips AD, Milla PJ, Bottazzo GF, Harries JT. Specific autoantibodies to gut epithelium in two infants with severe protracted diarrhoea. J Pediatr Gastroenterol Nutr 1985;4:187-195.

COELIAC DISEASE, MALIGNANCY AND THE EFFECT OF GLUTEN FREE DIET.

G.K.T. Holmes, MD, FRCP. Derbyshire Royal Infirmary, Derby, UK.

The most serious complication of coeliac disease (CD) is the development of malignancy, particularly lymphoma, which at presentation is usually widespread and the prognosis is correspondingly very poor. Earlier diagnosis of malignancy would improve the outlook for patients, but this poses difficulties which are unlikely to be surmounted in the near future. The question then arises: can this complication be prevented or reduced by strict adherence to a gluten free diet (GFD)?.
A long-term study of 210 patients with CD seen in the Gastrointestinal Unit at the General Hospital Birmingham was set up to try and answer this question. The initial review of these patients at the end of 1974 confirmed the high occurrence of malignancy among the group, but could not demonstrate that a GFD prevented this complication, probably because the time on diet was relatively short. This same series was kept under surveillance to document any further cancers and to further assess the effects of a GFD on the development of malignancy during more prolonged follow-up. The patients were reviewed at the end of 1985 - after 11 more years of observation. Twelve new cancers occurred, of which one was a carcinoma of the oesophagus and two lymphomas. In total thirty nine cancers developed in 38 patients and of 69 deaths, 33 were the result of malignancy. A two-fold relative risk of cancer was found and was because of an increased risk of cancer of the mouth and pharynx, oesophagus and non-Hodgkin's lymphoma.
The results indicate that the risk of developing cancer over all sites is not increased compared with the general population for coeliac patients who have taken a GFD for five consecutive years or more. The risk is increased, however, for those taking a reduced gluten diet or a normal diet, with a significant excess of cancers of the mouth, pharynx and oesophagus and of lymphoma. A significant decreasing trend in excess morbidity over increasing use of a GFD was found. Forty years ago Dicke and his colleagues established the value of the GFD in restoring the health of patients with CD. The results from the present study support a protective role for the GFD with regard to malignancy complicating the disorder and is a further reason for advising all patients to adhere to a strict diet for life. These observations extend even further the value of the GFD in the management of CD.

INTRODUCTION

The early literature of malabsorption which has recently been reviewed (1), records that patients often died of malignancy, particularly lymphoma. In the reports up to 1961, the malabsorption in every case was considered to occur secondary to the lymphoma. In 1962 however, Gough (2) from Bristol suggested that lymphoma is a complication of CD and that the mucosal lesion in this disorder is a premalignant condition. The hypothesis was strengthened by a further publication from this group (3) while at the same time evidence from Birmingham was also supportive (4). The researchers in Birmingham surveyed 202 patients with CD or idiopathic steatorrhoea

M. L. Mearin and C. J. J. Mulder (eds.), Coeliac Disease, 137–145.

and in addition to an increased prevalence of lymphoma, also found an increased risk of gastrointestinal carcinoma in general and oesophageal carcinoma in particular. Others have confirmed the association. Whorwell (5) found 31 of 77 deaths among members of the Coeliac Society of the United Kingdom to be due to malignancy and of these 10 resulted from lymphoma. In a series of 74 coeliac patients diagnosed in Sweden between 1965 and 1977, five (7%) developed lymphoma (6). In Galway, an area with a high prevalence of CD, 16 patients with malignant complications were seen between 1969 and 1981, of whom 10 had lymphoma. During these years 198 coeliac patients over the age of 12 years were diagnosed so the proportion who developed malginancy was 8% (7). Selby and Gallagher (8) recognised malignancy in 10 of 93 patients (11%) seen between 1958 and 1978. Five of these had oesophageal cancer and four lymphoma. In a further series of 100 patients followed for 18 years, malignancy was confirmed in eight and suspected in another 3 (9). When the Birmingham series originally reported by Harris and his colleagues was re-investigated in 1975, 11 more patients had developed malignancies of which 4 were lymphomas, making 18 (9%) for the whole group over the years out of a total of 43 cancers, an incidence of 21% (10). One puzzle was why cancer of the upper small bowel should appear to be so unusual, especially as this is the part of the intestine most abnormal in CD. A British collaborative study of CD which reported in 1983 however, showed that this malignancy is the second commonest after lymphoma, which illustrates the great value of pooling information from many centres when uncommon occurrences are being investigated (11).

THE DIFFICULTIES OF DIAGNOSIS OF MALIGNANCY IN COELIAC DISEASE.

The diagnosis of lymphoma complicating CD is difficult and may be delayed because the presenting features are often non-specific and indistinguishable from uncomplicated CD in relapse perhaps because of departure from a strict GFD. In most patients the tumour is widely disseminated at diagnosis and the prognosis is correspondingly very poor. In a third of cases in one series, the diagnosis was only made at autopsy (12). Unexplained deterioration in a coeliac patient previously well controlled on a GFD is a cause for concern and the development of weight loss, muscle weakness, pyrexia and lymphadenopathy should always raise the suspicion of lymphoma. The newly diagnosed adult patient requires careful observation for among one group, one in 20 had developed lymphoma within 4 years of the diagnosis of CD. Over the age of 50 years the risk was one in 10 (13).

While patients with lymphoma complicating CD are unable to maintain normal haematological and biochemical indices there is no pattern of abnormality which enables lymphoma to be diagnosed early. A progressive rise in serum IgA is sometimes seen which led to speculation that this might herald the onset of lymphoma but this observation is of limited value as raised levels may be found in CD without malignancy (14). Increased levels of lysozyme have been found in malignant histocytosis but are not a reliable indicator of lymphoma in CD (15-17). Changes in the inflammatory cell infiltrate of the small intestinal mucosa have been described in those patients who eventually develop malignancy which differ from those who do not (18). These consist of lower plasma cell and higher lymphocyte counts in the lamina propria and lower lymphocyte counts in the epithelium compared with biopsies from untreated coeliac patients. Comment has also been made on the presence of hypoplastic crypts (19) and histiocytic aggregates (20). However, prospective studies have never been mounted and these observations, even if true, are unlikely to be helpful in the individual case. Similar criticism can be made of trying to make an early diagnosis of lymphoma by measuring the response of blood lymphocytes to phytohaemagglutinin (21). Upper gastrointestinal endoscopy has the potential to diagnose early lesions (22) but other techniques, including computed tomography, appear to have nothing to offer in this regard. Bowel radiology may be normal in advanced disease and it may be necessary to resort to laparotomy when suspicion of malignancy is high and other avenues have failed to make a firm diagnosis (12). When cancer is found, it is usually widespread, although occasionally a curative resection is possible, especially when a localised bowel lymphoma or a stenosing carcinoma of the small intestine is found (23).

CAN A GFD REDUCE MALIGNANCY IN COELIAC DISEASE?

It is clear that the early diagnosis of malignancy in CD still poses formidable difficulties which are unlikely to be surmounted in the near future. The question then arises, can this complication be prevented or reduced by strict adherence to a GFD? Some considerations suggest that this might be so. The jejunal mucosa in CD has features of premalignancy with regard to both carcinoma (24) and lymphoma (2). These include increased mitotic activity in the crypts and lymphoid cells and irregularity and increased basophilia of the surface epithelium. Carcinogens may more easily penetrate the damaged mucosa which may also be deficient in carcinogen detoxifying enzymes (25). A GFD substantially restores the architecture of the mucosa towards normal and may therefore, also reduce the malignant potential.

A LONG TERM STUDY OF MALIGNANCY AND THE EFFECTS OF A GFD IN 210 PATIENTS WITH COELIAC DISEASE.

Review at the end of 1974: in order to investigate malignancy and CD further and particularly to try and determine whether a GFD reduces the malignant potential, a study of 210 patients seen in the Gastrointestinal Unit at the General Hospital Birmingham up to the end of 1972 and followed to the end of 1974 were reviewed (10). A statistically significant increase in deaths from cancer occurred in the whole series and in men and women separately. An increase was noted in deaths from lymphoma in men and women separately and in oesophageal and pharyngeal cancer in men (Table I). Unfortunately it could not be demonstrated that a GFD was effective in preventing these complications. Patients who had taken the diet for less than 12 months were grouped with those who had been having a conventional diet. All who had been treated for longer than 12 months with a GFD were considered together irrespective of their clinical response. In both groups there was an excess of deaths from all malignancies and lymphomas when compared with the general population (Table II). A further analysis of the data revealed that seven tumors occurred in those patients who had taken the diet for longer than one year, a figure significantly in excess of that expected, all in subjects who had shown a good clinical response to gluten withdrawal. Deaths from lymphoma in those on a normal diet and in those treated with a GFD were also significantly increased. These findings were perhaps not surprising if protection is dependant on the duration and strictness of a GFD, as the average time on diet was only 7.5 years.

TABLE I DEATHS DUE TO MALIGNANCY AMONG 210 PATIENTS WITH COELIAC DISEASE

Group	Observed	Expected	P
Total group (210)			
All malignancies	21	5.048	$p<0.001$
Reticulum cell sarcoma	13	0.114	$p<0.001$
Ca oesophagus	2	0.098	$p<0.01$
Ca pharynx	2	0.027	$p<0.001$
Men (94)			
All malignancies	12	2.878	$p<0.001$
Reticulum cell sarcoma	6	0.062	$p<0.001$
Ca oesophagus	2	0.053	$p<0.01$
Ca pharynx	2	0.013	$p<0.001$
Women (116)			
All malignancies	9	2.170	$p<0.001$
Reticulum cell sarcoma	7	0.052	$p<0.001$
Ca oesophagus	0	0.045	NS
CA pharynx	0	0.014	NS

Review at the end of 1985: this same series was kept under surveillance to document any further cancers and to further assess the effects of a GFD on the development of malignancy during more prolonged follow-up. The patients were reviewed at the end of 1985 i.e. after 11 more years of observation (26). Of the 69 deaths which had occurred, 33 were due to malignancy and overall there were 39 cancers in 38 patients. For this new review, which included living and dead patients with malignancy, the cases were re-evaluated so that a better analysis could be carried out than was previously achieved. The analysis at the and of 1974 included eight patients, all dead, in whom the interval between the diagnosis of CD and malignancy was one year or less. These patients are of interest and many observations strengthen the view that they should be regarded as having CD complicated by malignancy (22). Nevertheless, for the 1985 review these were excluded from statistical consideration because the development of malignancy was the event which led to the diagnosis of CD and could be a potential source of bias in the analysis. This re-evaluation which included other minor changes allowed 19 patients to be included in the analysis as having developed malignancy up to the end of 1974. From the end 1974 to the end of 1985, 12 new cancers occurred and since one patient had two malignancies, for the whole series there were 31 tumours among 30 patients. For the whole group of 210 patients the male: female ratio was 1:1.2, the men contributing a mean of 17.4 person-years at risk and the women 19.4 years. The minimum possible follow up was 13 years (end of 1974 to the end of 1985). The analysis compared cancer morbidity in the series with that in the general population using the method of years at risk and the expected numbers of tumours calculated and compared with those observed.

TABLE II DEATHS FROM MALIGNANCY IN COELIAC DISEASE RELATED TO DIETARY HISTORY

Group	No	Observed	Expected	P
All malignancies				
All GFD	134	7	1.259	$p<0.001$
ND	76	14	3.790	$p<0.001$
Retic cell sarc				
All GFD	134	4	0.038	$p<0.001$
ND	76	9	0.760	$p<0.001$
Ca oesophagus				
All GFD	134	1	0.030	$p<0.05$
ND	76	1	0.067	NS
Ca pharynx				
All GFD	134	1	0.007	$p<0.01$
ND	76	1	0.020	$p<0.05$

GFD =patients treated with a gluten free diet for longer than one year irrespective of the clinical response. ND =patients taking a normal diet plus those treated with a gluten free diet for less than one year.

Cancers at the end of 1985: a two-fold relative risk of cancer was found in the series (Table III), the differences between the observed and expected numbers being highly significant (RR=2.0, $P<0.001$). The excess was because of increased risk of cancers of the mouth, pharynx, oesophagus and of non-Hodgkin's lymphoma. No other individual sites showed an excess risk and the relative risks for cancer of the mouth and pharynx and for the oesophagus were similar being 9.7 and 12.3 respectively. The confidence intervals were wide but showed a lower limit of about 2.0 for both sites. All three oesophageal cancers were squamous cell tumours. A highly significant excess of non-Hodgkin's lymphoma was evident (RR=42.7, $p<0.001$). The lower limit for the confidence intervals was 20 fold.

TABLE III CANCER MORBIDITY IN 210 PATIENTS WITH COELIAC DISEASE AT THE END OF 1985

Site of cancer	ICD 8	Obs	Exp	O/E	P
All sites	140-208	31	15.48	2.0	p<0.001
Mouth and pharynx	140-147	3	0.31	9.7	p<0.01
Oesophagus	150	3	0.24	12.3	p<0.01
Non-Hodgkin's lymphoma	200-202	9	0.21	42.7	p<0.001
G I Tract	151-154	3	3.07	1.0	NS
Remainder		13	11.65	1.1	NS

Cancer arising 1975-1985: during these years a further 12 cancers occurred (Table IV). For the three sites mouth and pharynx, oesophagus and lymphoma 0.40 malignancies were expected (RR=7.5, p<0.01).

TABLE IV OCCURRENCE OF MALIGNANCY TO THE END OF 1974 AND FROM THE END OF 1974 TO THE END OF 1985

Site of cancer	31-12-1974 Obs	Exp	O/E	P
All sites	19	7.38	2.6	p<0.001
Mouth and pharynx	3	0.16	19.4	p<0.001
Oesophagus	2	0.11	18.7	p<0.01
Non-Hodgkin's lymphoma	7	0.10	67.3	p<0.001
Remainder	7	7.01	1.0	-
	01-01-1975 to 31-12-1985			
All sites	12	8.10	1.5	-
Mouth and pharynx	0	0.16	-	-
Oesophagus	1	0.13	7.5	-
Non-Hodgkin's lymphoma	2	0.11	18.9	p<0.01
Remainder	9	7.66	1.2	-

Cancers in relation to a GFD: the series was divided into three groups to reflect exposure to gluten.

1 Strict GFD group: patients who had kept to a strict GFD for five or more consecutive years. The five year period was an arbitrary decision before the analyses were carries out. This criterion was satisfied by 108 patients.
2 Normal diet group: a group of 46 patients had not taken a GFD.
3 Reduced gluten diet: this group of 56 patients included 17 who had taken diet for less than five years and 39 who had taken it spasmodically so that gluten free years could not properly be evaluated.

The normal diet group and the reduced gluten group showed little difference with regard to relative risks and because of the small numbers in the groups, for most of the analyses these have been combined and designated Group 2 and compared with Group 1, the strict GFD group as defined above.

When the groups were analysed separately (Table V), the risk of cancer over all sites was not significantly increased for the "strict GFD group" (Group 1). The risk was increased in those taking a reduced or a normal diet (Group 2). The small excess in Group 1 was accounted for mainly by the occurence of two non-Hodgkin's lymphomas. Patients having a normal or reduced gluten intake showed an excess of cancers of the mouth, pharynx and oesophagus and of lymphoma. Although no differences could be detected between the groups for individual sites, on combining them (mouth, pharynx, oesophagus and lymphoma), the difference between the relative risks - 6.7 for Group 1 and 38.6 for Group 2 - was statistically significant ($P<0.05$). When the groups were put into the three original diet groups, a significant decreasing trend in excess morbidity rate (EMR) over increasing use of a GFD was found (Table VI).

TABLE V CANCER MORBIDITY BY DIET GROUP

Site	Diet group	N	Obs	Exp	O/E	P
All sites	1	108	14	9.06	1.5	-
	2	102	17	6.42	2.6	p<0.001
Mouth, pharynx, oesophagus	1	108	1	0.33	3.0	-
	2	102	5	0.22	22.7	p<0.001
Non-Hodgkin's lymphoma	1	108	2	0.12	16.7	p<0.01
	2	102	7	0.09	77.8	p<0.001
Remainder	1	108	11	8.61	1.3	-
	2	102	5	6.11	0.8	-

TABLE VI CANCER MORBIDITY BY THREE DIET GROUPS IN MOUTH, PHARYNX, OESOPHAGUS AND LYMPHOMA

Group	N	Obs	Exp	O/E	P	EMR/10^3 PYR
Normal diet	46	7	0.19	36.8	p<0.001	10.7
Reduced gluten	56	5	0.12	41.7	p<0.001	5.0
Strict GFD	108	3	0.46	6.5	p<0.05	1.2

Trend for EMR over diet group: $X^2 = 9.9$; $p < 0.01$; EMR = excess morbidity rate (O - E / PYR x 10^3)

CONCLUSION

In 1950, Dicke (27) clearly demonstrated that the removal of wheat from the diet caused the symptoms and signs of CD to disappear and he had his colleagues extended these observations over the next few years in a classic series of experiments which firmly established the value of the GFD in restoring the health of patients. The results from the present study support a protective role for the GFD with regard to malignancy in CD and is a further reason for advising all patients to adhere to a strict diet for life. These observations extend even further the value of the GFD in the management of CD.

REFERENCES

1 Cooke WT, Holmes GKT. Malignancy. In: Coeliac Disease. Edinburgh. Churchill Livingstone. 1984.
2 Gough KR, Read AE, Naish JM. Intestinal reticulosis as a complication of idiopathic steatorrhoea. Gut 1967;3:232-239.
3 Austad WI, Cornes JS, Gough KR, McCarthy CF, Read AE. Steatorrhoea and malignant lymphoma. The relationship of malignant tumours of lymphoid tissue and coeliac disease. Am J of Dig Dis 1967;12:475-490.
4 Harris OD, Cooke WT, Thompson H, Waterhouse JAH. Malignancy in adult coeliac disease and idiopathic steatorrhoea. Am J of Med 1967;42:899-912.
5 Whorwell PJ, Foster KJ, Alderson MR, Wright R. Death from ischaemic heart disease and malignancy in adult coeliac disease. Lancet 1976;2:113-114.
6 Brandt L, Hagander B, Norden A, Stenstam M. Lymphoma of the small intestine in adult coeliac disease. Acta Med Scand 1978;204:467-470.
7 O'Driscoll BRC, Stevens FM, O'Gorman TA, Finnegan P, McWeeney JJ, Little MPG, Connolly CE, McCArthy CF. HLA type of patients with coeliac disease and malignancy in the West of Ireland. Gut 1982;23:662-665.
8 Selby WS, Gallagher ND. Malignancy in a 19 year experience of adult coeliac disease. Dig Dis Sci 1979;24:684-688.
9 Nielsen OH, Jacobsen O, Pederson ER, Rasmussen SN, Petri M, Laulund S, Jarnum S. Non-tropical sprue. Malignant diseases and mortality rate. Scand J of Gastroenterol 1985;20:13-18.
10 Holmes GKT, Stokes PL, Sorahan TM, Prior P, Waterhouse JAH, Cooke WT. Coeliac disease, gluten free diet and malignancy. Gut 1976;17:612-619.
11 Swinson CM, Slavin G, Coles EC, Booth CC. Coeliac disease and malignancy. Lancet 1983;1:111-115.
12 Cooper BT, Holmes GKT, Ferguson R, Cooke WT. Coeliac disease and malignancy. Medicine 1980;59:249-261.
13 Cooper BT, Holmes GKT, Cooke WT. Lymphoma risk in coeliac disease of later life. Digestion 1982;23:89-92.
14 Asquith P, Thompson RA, Cooke WT. Serum immunoglobulins in adult coeliac disease. Lancet 1969;2:129-131.
15 Hodges JR, Isaacson P, Eade OE, Wright R. Serum lysozyme levels in malignant histiocytosis of the intestine. Gut 1979;20:854-857.
16 Cooper BT, Ukabam SO, Barry RE, Read AE. Serum lysozyme activity in coeliac disease: a possible aid to the diagnosis of malignant change? J Clin Path 1981;34:1358-1360.
17 Bourke MA, McLoughlin DM, Stevens FM, Mc.Carthy CF. Serum lysozyme: is it a useful marker of malignant lymphoma in coeliac disease. Ir J of Med Sci 1983;152:125-128.
18 Ferguson R, Asquith P, Cooke WT. The jejunal cellular infiltrate in coeliac disease complicated by lymphoma. Gut 1974;15:458-461.
19 Barry RE, Read AE. Coeliac disease and malignancy. Quart J of Med 1973;42:665-675.
20 Isaacson P. Malignant histiocytosis of the intestine: the early histological lesion. Gut 1980;21:381-386.

21 Stenstam M, Brandt L, Hallberg T. Subnormal responses of blood lymphocytes to phytohaemagglutinin in adult coeliac disease complicated by intestinal lymphoma. Scand J of Gastroenterol 1983;18:777-781.
22 Cooper BT, Read AE. Coeliac disease and lymphoma. Quart J of Med 1987;63:269-274.
23 Holmes GKT, Dunn GI, Cockel R, Brookes VS. Adenocarcinoma of the upper small bowel complicating coeliac disease. Gut 1980;21:1010-1016.
24 Joske RA. Primary carcinoma of the jejunum with atrophic jejunitis and intestinal malabsorption. Gastroenterology 1960;38:810-816.
25 Wattenberg LW. Carcinogen detoxifying mechanisms in the gastrointestinal tract. Gastroenterology 1966;51:932-935.
26 Holmes GKT, Prior P, Lane MR, Pope P, Allan RN. Malignancy in coeliac disease - effect of a gluten free diet. Gut 1989;30:333-338.
27 Dicke WK. 1950. Coeliac disease; investigation of the harmful effects of certain types of cereal on patients with coeliac disease. Doctoral Thesis, University of Utrecht.

DERMATITIS HERPETIFORMIS: COELIAC DISEASE OF THE SKIN.

Timo Reunala, Dept. of Dermatology and Clinical Sciences, University of Tampere, SF-33520 Tampere, Finland.

Dermatitis herpetiformis (DH) is characterized by intense itch and small blisters with predilection sites on elbows, knees and buttocks. The diagnosis of DH is easy because all patients have pathognomonic IgA deposits in the papillary dermis of both involved and uninvolved skin. Patients with DH rarely present with GI symptoms although at least 80% of them have jejunal villous atrophy. Gluten loading causes villous atrophy in the remaining patients showing that also these patients are sensitive to gluten. Interestingly, also the rash responds to gluten withdrawal and relapses on gluten challenge and therefore, a life-long gluten-free diet (GFD) is now the treatment of choice for all patients with DH. The present clinical evidence shows that the skin-gut relationship is very close in DH but the pathomechanism of the rash remains open. IgA disapppears rarely from the skin during GFD treatment, and all efforts to show gluten in the skin or to characterize the antigen for IgA have failed. Immunogenetic and family studies have produced further evidence that DH seems to be only a specific skin manifestation of coeliac disease. The HLA pattern in DH is similar to that reported in coeliac disease and DH patients seem to have as often affected relatives as patients with coeliac disease (CD). In our series of 776 DH patients we found 78 (10%) with affected first-degree relatives. The disease encountered in these relatives was in addition to DH often also coeliac disease. Of the 28 affected sibpairs 14 were DH-coeliac disease and 14 DH-DH pairs, and most of these pairs were concordant for HLA haplotype B8, DR3. We have found also two DH-DH couples whose children have no evidence for DH but have conctracted coeliac disease.

INTRODUCTION

DH is an intensely itchy, chronic papulovesicular skin disorder. The definitive diagnosis is made by skin immunofluorescence examination which shows pathognomonic granular IgA deposits in the upper dermis. The nature and origin of these immunoglobulin deposits remain unknown. Essentially all DH patients have subclinical gluten-sensitive enteropathy and the rash responds to strict GFD treatment showing that gluten plays a central role in the pathophysiology of DH. Recent immunogenetic and family data further support the view that DH is a specific skin manifestation of CD.

CLINICAL PRESENTATION AND PREVALENCE

Characteristically the papulovesicular lesions are symmetrically distributed on the elbows, knees, buttocks and upper back. Early lesions are often excoriated due to intense pruritus and scratching; occasionally larger blisters can be seen. The intensity of the rash varies from very mild to severe from patient to patient. Spontaneous remissions are very infrequent in patients with more active disease (1,2). The mean

M. L. Mearin and C. J. J. Mulder (eds.), Coeliac Disease, 147–151.

age at onset is 30-35 years (fig.1) but DH can start in childhood or even appear after the age of 70 years (2,3). In contrast to CD, males contract DH more often than females (2). The prevalence of DH seems to vary with the ethnicity of populations. Prevalences of 1/2000 to 1/10.000 have been reported in Finland, Sweden and Scotland but patients with DH are rarely seen in Japan (2,4-6). In countries with frequent occurrence of DH, the prevalence is about 1/2-1/5 of that of CD (7,8).

FIGURE I AGE AT ONSET OF DERMATITIS HERPETIFORMIS IN 345 FINNISH PATIENTS

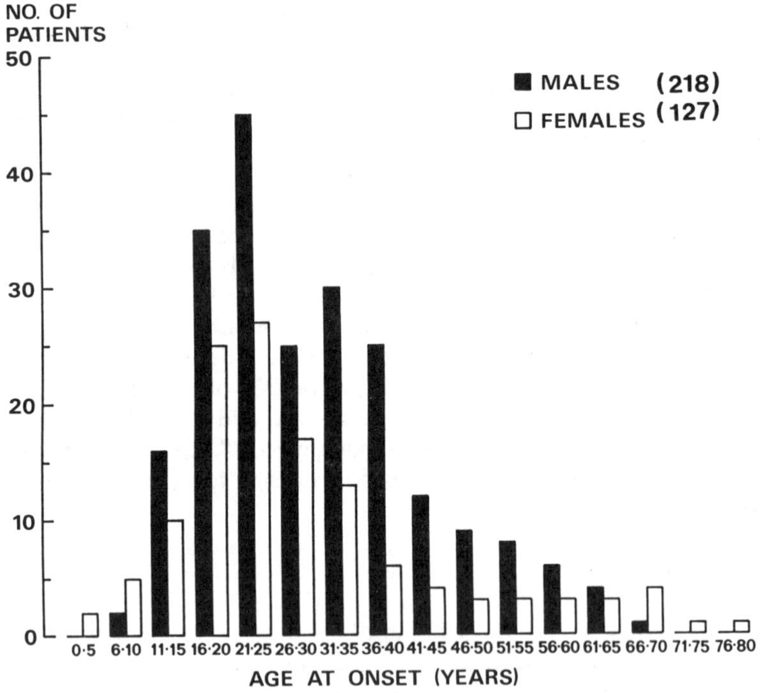

SMALL INTESTINE IN DERMATITIS HERPETIFORMIS

The association of DH with CD was first discovered in 1966 by Marks (9). The degree of jejunal villous atrophy can be variable, but at least 70%-80% of the patients show subtotal or partial villous atrophy in a single jejunal biopsy. Multiple biopsies have shown that the mucosal lesion can be patchy in some DH patients (2). The remaining patients with normal villous architecture often show increased intra-epithelial lymphocyte counts and increased numbers of IgA-bearing lymphocytes in lamina propria (10,11). Moreover, gluten loading can be used to produce pathological changes in at least some of the patients with normal villous architecture (12). Further evidence of the existence of dose-dependent gluten-sensitive enteropathy in DH was reported by Andersson (13). They found in 36 DH patients that the mean daily intake of gluten varied from 4 to 26 grams and that patients with villous atrophy consumed significantly higher amounts of gluten than those having normal jejunal mucosa. It is, however, difficult to explain why gluten-sensitive enteropathy is mostly subclinical in patients with DH. Only a few patients have G-I symptoms and laboratory findings of malabsorption occur only in 10%-20% of the patients (3,10).

EFFECT OF GLUTEN-FREE DIET

There is now general agreement that the rash responds to gluten withdrawal (14). After adhering to GFD most DH patients can reduce the dosage of dapsone, a sulfone drug needed to control their cutaneous lesions when they are following a normal gluten-containing diet. After two years or longer on a GFD up to 70% of the patients can control their skin disease completely without drugs (1,2,15). The success of the GFD treatment in DH seems to be directly related to compliance alone and the rash reponds similarly to diet both in patients with and without jejunal villous atrophy (15). Usually the skin and gut response to GFD parallel each other, and the rash clears up although some abnormalities, such as increased intraepithelial lymphocyte counts, persist in the small intestine (1,2,11).

The reason for the incomplete skin response to GFD may be the continuous intake of small amounts of gluten (14). It is also puzzling that at the beginning of the diet treatment the rash may recur in some patients even after intake of minute amounts of gluten, such as drinking two bottles of beer. After several asymptomatic years on a GFD it takes longer before the rash recurs on gluten challenge. Leonard (16) observed a recurrence in 11 of their 12 adult patients with DH after an average interval of 3 months on gluten challenge. Similar relapses occur in children with DH challenged with gluten, and in these patients the reappearance of the rash has been shown to parallel the deterioration of the small intestinal lesion (3,11). Therefore, the current evidence both in children and adults with DH indicates that GFD treatment needs to be continued indefinitely.

The presence of IgA in the skin of patients with DH has led to the hypothesis that the IgA may originate from the gut as a result of immune response to gluten or other dietary antigens. However, the specificity of IgA is still obscure. The antibody subclass is mainly A1, and there is no evidence of any unique antigen to which IgA antibody binds in the skin (17,18). Cutaneous IgA deposits appear to be resistant to GFD treatment. They persist in the uninvolved skin even though the rash has cleared, and only two groups of investigators have documented the disappearance of IgA deposits (16,19). This occurred in only a few DH patients after they had been totally asymptomatic for several years on a strict GFD. When these patients with negative immunofluorescence findings have been challenged with gluten, IgA has reappeared before or at the same time as the rash suggesting that IgA deposition is also a gluten-dependent phenomenon in DH (16).

IMMUNOGENETICS AND FAMILY STUDIES

The response of the skin lesions to gluten withdrawal is one of the most compelling pieces of evidence linking DH to CD. Immunogenetic and family data provide further evidence of this linkage. About 90% of the patients with DH and CD have

HLA class II antigen DR3 and an even stronger association has been found with DQw2 (20,21). Sachs (20) also found an increased frequency of DR2 in DH and suggested that this antigen is important for the development of skin disease. Hall (21) could not confirm this and therefore, the hypothesis for the different HLA DR gene contributions in DH and CD seems not to be valid.

The recent evidence from restriction fragment polymorphism analysis suggests that the primary HLA association could be with certain HLA DQ α/β genes in CD and it remains to be seen whether the same genes occur in patients with DH (22).

The familial incidence of CD is 10%-20% (23). Several recent surveys have brought evidence that also DH is a familiar disease. In Utah, Meyer and Zone (24) found in a series of 92 DH patients that six (6.5%) of them had first-degree relatives who were affected. In Ireland, Love (25) observed that 2.5% of the 446 relatives of his DH patients were affected. In the Finnish DH series of 530 patients followed-up for several years 24 (4.5%) patients had first-degree relatives with DH and interestingly, 29 (5.5%) patients had relatives with CD (26). Of the 28 sibling pairs 14 were DH-DH pairs and 14 were DH-CD pairs showing that clinical CD occurs as frequently as DH in relatives of Finnish patients with DH.

The reports on affected monozygotic twins provide important additional evidence that DH seems to be only a specific skin manifestation of CD. Four twin pairs have been reported in literature; two of them have been concordant for DH, the other two pairs had one twin with DH and the other with CD (27-30). The Finnish DH series consists of three affected monozygotic twins; one pair is concordant for DH, the other two pairs are discordant (T. Reunala, unpublished observation). The monozygotic twin data showing discordance for DH but concordance for CD obviously indicate that some non-genetic factors are important for the development of skin disease, i.e. DH, in people having a genetically determined gluten-sensitive enteropathy.

REFERENCES

1 Fry L, Leonard JN, Swain F et al. Long term follow-up of dermatitis herpetiformis with and without dietary gluten withdrawal. British Journal of Dermatology 1982;107:631-640.

2 Gawkrodger DJ, Blackwell JN, Gilmour HM et al. Dermatitis herpetiformis: diagnosis, diet and demography. Gut 1984;25:151-157.

3 Reunala T, Kosnai I, Karpati S et al. Dermatitis herpetiformis: jejunal findings and skin response to gluten free diet. Archives of Diseases in Childhood 1984;59:517-522.

4 Reunala T & Lokki J. Dermatitis herpetiformis in Finland. Acta Dermato-Venereologica 1978;58:505-510.

5 Hashimoto K, Miki Y, Nishioka K et al. HLA antigens in dermatitis herpetiformis among Japanese. Journal of Dermatology 1980;7:289-291.

6 Moi H. Incidence and prevalence of dermatitis herpetiformis in a county of central Sweden. Acta Dermato-Venereologica 1984;64:144-150.

7 Hallert C, Gotthard K, Norrby K & Walan A. On the prevalence of adult coeliac disease in Sweden. Scandinavian Journal of Gastroenterology 1981;16:257-261.

8 Logan RFA, Rifkind EA, Busuttil A et al. Prevalence and incidence of celiac disease in Edinburg and the Lothian region of Scotland. Gastroenterology 1986;90:334-342.

9 Marks J, Shuster S & Watson AJ. Small bowel changes in dermatitis herpetiformis. Lancet 1966;2:1280.

10 Katz SI, Hall RP, Lawley TJ & Strober W. Dermatitis herpetiformis: the skin and the gut. Annals of Internal Medicine 1980;93:857-874.

11 Kosnai I, Karpati S, Savilahti E et al. Gluten challenge in children with dermatitis herpetiformis: a clinical, morphological and immunohistological study. Gut 1986;27:1464-1470.
12 Ferguson A, Blackwell JN & Barnetson RStC. Effects of additional dietary gluten on the small-intestinal mucosa of volunteers and of patients with dermatitis herpetiformis. Scandinavian Journal of Gastroenterology 1987;22:543-549.
13 Andersson H, Björkman A-C, Gillberg R et al. Influence of the amount of dietary gluten on gastrointestinal morphology and function in dermatitis herpetiformis. Human Nutrition and Clinical Nutrition 1984;38:279-285.
14 Hall RP. Dietary management of dermatitis herpetiformis. Archives of Dermatology 1987;123:1378a-1380a.
15 Reunala T, Blomqvist K, Tarpila S et al. Gluten free diet in dermatitis herpetiformis. I. Clinical response of skin lesions in 81 patients. British Journal of Dermatology 1977;97:473-480.
16 Leonard JN, Haffenden G, Tucker W et al. Gluten challenge in dermatitis herpetiformis. New England Journal of Medicine 1983;308:816-819.
17 Egelrud T & Bäck O. Dermatitis herpetiformis: biochemical properties of the granular deposits of IgA in papillary dermis. Journal of Investigative Dermatology 1985;84:239-245.
18 Kadunce DP, Meyer LJ & Zone JJ. IgA class antibodies in dermatitis herpetiformis: reaction with tissue antigens. Journal of Investigative Dermatology 1989;93:253-258.
19 Reunala T & Salo OP. Effects of long-term gluten-free diet in dermatitis herpetiformis. In Kukita A and Seiji M (eds) Proceedings of the XVI International Congress of Dermatology 1983; pp.411-413, Tokyo: University of Tokyo Press.
20 Sachs JA, Awad J, McCloskey D et al. Different HLA associated gene combinations contribute to susceptibility for coeliac disease and dermatitis herpetiformis. Gut 1986;27:515-520.
21 Hall RP, Sanders ME, Duquesnoy RJ et al. Alterations in HLA-DP and HLA- DQ antigen frequency in patients with dermatitis herpetiformis. Journal of Investigative Dermatology 1989;93:501-505.
22 Sollid LM, Markussen G, Ek J et al. Evidence for a primary association of celiac disease to a particular HLA-DQ α/β heterodimer. Journal of Experimental Medicine 1989;169:345-350.
23 Cooke WT & Holmes GKT. Coeliac Disease 1984; pp.17-19. Edinburg: Churchill Livingstone.
24 Meyer LJ & Zone JJ. Familial incidence of dermatitis herpetiformis. Journal of American Academy of Dermatology 1987;17:643-647.
25 Love AHG. Epidemiological and genetic aspects of the coeliac syndrome in relation to dermatitis herpetiformis. In McConnell RB (ed) The Genetics of Coeliac Disease 1981; pp.95-99. Lancaster: MTP Press.
26 Reunala T, Karvonen J & Koskimies S. Dominant inheritance of dermatitis herpetiformis. In Orfanos CE et al (eds) Abstracts of the 17th World Congress of Dermatology 1987; II, p.289, Berlin: University Medical Center Steglitz.
27 Marks J, May SB & Roberts DF. Dermatitis herpetiformis occurring in monozygotic twins. British Journal of Dermatology 1971;84:417-419.
28 Jepsen LV & Ullman S. Dermatitis herpetiformis and gluten-sensitive enteropathy in monozygotic twins. Acta Dermato-Venereologica 1980;60:353-355.
29 Kosnai I, Karpati S, Török E et al. Dermatitis herpetiformis in monozygotic twins: discordance for dermatitis herpetiformis and concordance for gluten-dose sensitive enteropathy. European Journal of Pediatrics 1985;144:404-405.
30 Green ST, Natarajan S, Connor JM & Forrest JAH. Monozygous twins concordant for duodenojejunal villous atrophy and dermatitis herpetiformis. Gut 1986;27:970-971.

LATENT COELIAC DISEASE.

M. Maki, K. Holm, S. Koskimies, J.K. Visakorpi. Department of Clinical Sciences, University of Tampere, 33520 Tampere, Finland.

We report four patients, two children, one adolescent and one adult having normal small-bowel mucosa on biopsy before the initial diagnosis of coeliac disease (CD) was made. The first biopsy was undertaken and found to be normal in two cases due to suspected malabsorption, in one due to suspected dermatitis herpetiformis and in one as part of a CD family study. After further 2.6 to 9 years on gluten-containing diet, small bowel villous atrophy with crypt hyperplasia compatible with CD was found. The HLA type of the patients was that typical for CD; all were DR3 positive. A closer look at the initial biopsies revealed minor pathology in an increased count of intraepithelial lymphocytes in two cases, but still with tall villous architecture. Hence they cannot be called CD patients and treated as such. We do not think mucosal patchiness explains the findings because the highly sensitive and specific antibody tests used by us (reticulin and endomysium) were negative at the time of the first biopsy and later positive when mucosal atrophy was manifest. Late-developing mucosal atrophy in CD (latent CD) may be much more common than previously assumed. This finding will change our conceptions of this condition. Also the understanding of the inheritance of CD must be re-evaluated.

INTRODUCTION

It is generally accepted that a normal small-bowel biopsy specimen, taken for the first time when the patient is eating normal gluten-containing food, rules out the diagnosis of CD once and for all. At present we demand an abnormal small-intestinal mucosa (subtotal villous atrophy or flat mucosa) as being essential for a diagnosis of CD. However, we have recently shown that CD may exist latent in patients having normal mucosa when eating a normal gluten-containing diet (1).

REVIEW OF LITERATURE

Late onset CD in the monozygotic twin of a coeliac child has been reported by both Kamath and Dorney (2) and Salazar de Sousa (3). This clearly indicates that CD may exist latent in patients having normal mucosa when eating a normal diet. There are a few more such patients described in the literature. McConnell and Whitwell (4) described a woman who at the age of 39 was biopsied because of suspected CD. Because of only mild partial villous atrophy the patient was judged not to have CD. Five years later she was again referred because of continuing diarrhoea and a second biopsy was carried out. On this occasion the jejunal mucosa showed total villous atrophy typical for CD. Polanco (5) report a boy with symptoms compatible with CD since the age of one year. He was found to have normal small-bowel villous architecture at the ages of two and three. At the age of 9 years subtotal villous atrophy was found and the mucosa normalized on gluten-free diet.
Rolles (6) biopsied a girl at the age of 4 years because of a vague history of ill

M. L. Mearin and C. J. J. Mulder (eds.), Coeliac Disease, 153–156.

health and a tenedency to loose motions and because the mother had one month earlier been diagnosed to have CD. A jejunal biopsy was entirely normal. At the mother's insistence she was reviewed two years later. The second biopsy was performed after adding extra gluten to the diet. No worsening of the symptoms was observed. The biopsy showed a completely flat mucosa and the child was put on a gluten-free diet. Freeman and Chiu (7) have shown that latent CD may be present in patients with malignant intestinal lymphoma. A 73 years old woman with resected jejunoileal lymphoma and normal proximal small-bowel biopsy specimens was given a high-gluten diet resulting in intestinal abnormalities typical for CD.

OWN PATIENTS

We have reported four patients, two children, one adolescent and one adult having normal small-bowel mucosa on biopsy before the initial diagnosis of CD was made (1). The first biopsy was undertaken and found to be normal in two cases due to suspected malabsorption, in one due to suspected dermatitis herpetiformis and in one as part of a CD family study. After a further 2.6 to 9 years on gluten-containing diet, small-bowel villous atrophy with crypt hyperplasia compatible with CD was found. The HLA type of the patients was that typical for CD; all were DR3 positive. A closer look at the initial biopsies revealed some pathology, but still with tall villous architecture (Table).

TABLE MORPHOMETRY OF NORMAL SMALL-BOWEL BIOPSIES AT THE LATENT STAGE OF CD.

Case number	IEL/100	Villus/crypt ratio
1	34	1.56
2	31	4.06
3	21	(>387)*
4	14	3.24

* Because of technical difficulties only villus height is given.

DISCUSSION

Our four cases are identical to those previously described in the literature (2-6); they were all first diagnosed to be free of CD and years later found to have the disease. A closer look at the initial biopsies revealed minor pathology in an increased count of intraepithelial lymphocytes in some cases, but still with tall villous architecture. Hence they cannot be called CD patients and treated as such. Low gluten intake may have influenced the villous architecture in two of the patients as there was in the family one earlier diagnosed case of CD on a gluten-free diet at the time of the first biopsy. In fact, it has been shown that low gluten diet has no significant effect on gross small-bowel mucosal architecture in CD (8). Another possible explanation is mucosal patchiness; flat mucosa might have been found even close to the biopsy site. However, we do not think this is a relevant explanation because the highly sensitive and specific antibody tests used by us (9,10) were negative at the time of the first biopsy and later positive when mucosal atrophy was manifest (1). Late-developing mucosal atrophy in CD (latent CD) may be much more common than previously assumed. Our results show that CD has not disappeared; the disease itself exists or appears late in the population even if classical forms disappear (11). Also in adults CD often presents itself with only mild or no abdominal symptoms (12, 13) and a greater awareness of the disease has led to an increasing number of cases diagnosed annually (14). Again in our family study about 10 % of first-degree relatives to CD patients was found to have symptomless CD (15). It is hardly possible that these patients have been asymptomatic with mucosal atrophy for decades; rather one would think that the disease with mucosal atrophy has developed late. In such cases an earlier mucosal biopsy would have shown normal villous architecture even if these CD patients had eaten normal amounts of gluten since early childhood. On the basis of the present study and the cases found in the literature it now seems that latent CD does exist. This is important in many respects, but especially true in the light of the possible development of malignancies in patients with untreated coeliac disease (16). This finding will change our conceptions of this condition. Also the understanding of the heredity of CD must be re-evaluated.

REFERENCES

1 Mäki M, Holm K, Koskimies S, Hällström O, Visakorpi JK. Normal small-bowel biopsy followed by coeliac disease. Arch Dis Child 1990;65:1137-41.

2 Kamath KR, Dorney SFA. Is discordance for coeliac disease in monozygotic twins permanent? Ped Res 1983;17:422.

3 Salazar de Sousa J, Ramos de Almeida JM, Monteiro MV, Magalhaes-Ramalho P. Late onset coeliac disease in the monozygotic twin of a coeliac child. Acta Paediatr Scand 1987;76:172-4.

4 McConnell RB, Whitwell F. Small-intestinal histology in coeliac disease. Lancet 1975;ii:418.

5 Polanco I, Larrauri J, Prieto G, Guerrero J, Pena AS, Vazquez C. Severe villous atrophy appearing at different ages in two coeliac siblings with identical HLA haplotypes. Acta Paediatr Belg 1980;33:276.

6 Rolles CJ, Kyaw-Myint TB, Wai-Kee Sin, Andersom CM. The familial incidence of asymptomatic coeliac disease. In: The Genetics of Coeliac Disease, McConnell RB ed., MTP Press Limited, International Medical Publishers, Lancaster- Boston- The Hague, 1981 p. 235-43.

7 Freeman HJ, Chiu BK. Multifocal small bowel lymphoma and latent celiac sprue. Gastroenterology 1986;90:1992-97.

8 Montgomery AMP, Goka AKJ, Kumar PJ, Farthing MJG, Clark ML. Low gluten diet in the treatment of adult coeliac disease: effect on jejunal morphology and serum anti-gluten antibodies. Gut 1988;29:1564-8.

9 Mäki M, Hällström O, Vesikari T, Visakorpi JK. Evaluation of a serum IgA-class reticulin antibody test for the detection of childhood celiac disease. Pediatr 1984;105:901-5.

10 Hällström O. Comparison of IgA-class reticulin and endomysium antibodies in coeliac disease and dermatitis herpetiformis. Gut 1989;30:1225-32.

11 Mäki M, Holm K. Incidence and prevalence of coeliac disease in Tampere. Coeliac disease is not disappearing. Acta Paediatr Scand 1990;79:980-82.

12 Swinson CM, Levi AJ. Is coeliac disease underdiagnosed? Br J Med 1980;281:1258-60.

13 Collin P, Hällström O, Mäki M, Viander M, Keyriläinen O. Atypical coeliac disease found with serological screening. Scand J Gastroenterol 1990;25:245-50.

14 Logan RFA, Tucker G, Rifkind EA, Heading RC, Ferguson A. Changes in clinical features of coeliac disease in adults in Edinburgh and the Lothians 1960-79. Br Med J 1983;286:95-7.
15 Auricchio S, Mazzacca G, Tosi R, Visakorpi J, Mäki M, Polanco I. Coeliac disease as a familial condition: Identification of asymptomatic coeliac patients within family groups. Gastroenterology International 1988;1:25-31.
16 Holmes GKT, Prior P, Lane MR, Pope D, Allan RN. Malignancy in coeliac disease - effect of a gluten free diet. Gut 1989;30:333-38.

SMALL INTESTINAL BIOPSY

H.S.A. Heymans*, J.F.W.M. Bartelsman, Dep.Paediatrics and Gastroenterology. Academic Medical Center Amsterdam, The Netherlands.
***Project Adress: Academic Hospital Groningen.**

Since its first description, some 34 years ago, peroral biopsy of the small intestine (SIB) has become and remained a valuable diagnostic procedure for small intestinal disorders. It has also substantially contributed to the understanding of the pathogenesis of diseases of the small intestinal mucosa. In childhood coeliac disease (CD) small intestinal biopsy is indispensable, as investigations of the jejunal mucosa at presentation, after gluten-free diet and after gluten-challenge, are still considered to be obligatory for definitive diagnosis. From 1980-1987 20 patients, suspected for CD on clinical and biochemical grounds, in which without a preceding investigation of the small intestinal mucosa a gluten-free diet was installed, have been referred to our department to confirm the diagnosis. In only 5 patients CD could be diagnosed by SIB before and after gluten-challenge. In 15 patients, with an average follow-up of 54 months, the diagnosis could not be confirmed. Installation of a glutenfree diet without indication can easily result in severe diagnostic delay and an unnecessary treatment of children with substantial psychological, social and financial consequences.

In recent years many investigators have tried to develop simpler, quicker and less traumatic tests to replace SIB, but so far no test has shown sufficient sensitivity and/or specificity. The importance of a reliable and effective diagnostic test has become increasingly important as epidemiological features seem to point out that the clinical picture of childhood CD is changing, involving older children with minor symptoms.

In an attempt to lower the threshold for a small intestinal biopsy and to improve the efficiency of this diagnostic procedure, a new technique has been developed within the Department of Pediatrics and Gastroenterology in the Academic Medical Center in Amsterdam. A pediatric biopsy capsule (Enraf Nonius) was connected to a hydraulic suction pump (Quinton) by two plastic tubes, one for hydraulic operation of the knife, and the other for flushing the mucosal specimen. To allow quick passage to the duodenal jejunal flexure a flexible iron guide wire is placed within one of the tubes before the capsule is advanced under fluoroscopic control.

In this way more than 250 pediatric and 1200 adult patients have been investigated during the last 8 years. In less than 1% of the patients the procedure was not succesful. The only complication was a severe bleeding in one adult patient, that stopped spontaneously. An average of 5 small intestinal biopsies per patient were available for investigation including routine histology, immuno-fluorescence, electron microscopy and biochemical investigation of brush border enzymes. After adequate preparation of the patient, including sedation in smaller pediatric patients, the procedure takes ± 15 minute per patient and can be performed on an outpatient basis. In our experience this technique has shown to be safe and efficient in the diagnosis of small intestinal disease. In our opinion, jejunal biopsies taken in this way are superior to endoscopic biopsies from the duodenum in diagnosing CD.

M. L. Mearin and C. J. J. Mulder (eds.), Coeliac Disease, 157–163.

INTRODUCTION

Since its first description, peroral biopsy of the small intestine has become and remained a valuable diagnostic procedure for small intestinal disorders (1,2). It has also substantially contributed to the understanding of the pathogenesis of diseases of the small intestinal mucosa. In coeliac disease (CD), investigation of the small intestinal mucosa is considered to be obligatory for definitive diagnosis (3-6). Initially the European Society of Pediatric Gastroenterology and Nutrition (ESPGAN) proposed the following diagnostic criteria:

- structural abnormal jejunum mucosa when taking a diet containing gluten;
- clear improvement of villus structure when taking a gluten-free diet;
- deterioration of the mucosa during gluten challenge (3,4).

Following these criteria three sequential small intestinal biopsies were necessary for differentiating CD from transient causes of abnormal small intestinal mucosa. However, re-evaluation of these criteria suggested that they might not invariably be requested for the diagnosis of all patients as the initial diagnosis made at the time of the first biopsy was confirmed in 619 out of 652 cases (95%) (5). Recently, revised criteria for the diagnosis of CD were reported by a working group of ESPGAN (6). A simplified diagnostic procedure was proposed in which the finding of a characteristic small intestinal mucosal abnormality on histological examination of a biopsy specimen was considered to be the first requirement of diagnosis. This together with a clear-cut clinical remission on strict glutenfree diet with release of all symptoms, was proposed to be sufficient for a definitive diagnosis of CD without requirement of gluten challenge. So even today small intestinal biopsy remains the cornerstone for the diagnosis of CD. It is generally accepted that no child should be placed on a glutenfree diet on the absence of characteristic abnormalities of the small intestinal mucosa on histological examination (7,8). However, Lloyd-Still (9) reported that 70% of the children referred to his institution for consultation because of chronic diarrhea, had been treated symptomatically with a glutenfree diet without the diagnosis been made. Such practice may complicate severely the diagnosis of CD.

PSEUDO-COELIAC DISEASE

From 1980-1987 20 patients, suspected for CD on clinical and biochemical grounds in which without a preceding investigation of the small intestinal mucosa a gluten free diet was installed, had been referred to one of the authors (HSAH) for confirmation of the diagnosis. All patients had been treated with a glutenfree diet for more than one year. Small bowel biopsies were performed before and after gluten challenge, confirming the diagnosis in only 5 patients. In the 15 remained patients a normal diet was installed. All 15 patients were free of symptoms during a follow-up of more than 3 years. These patients had been treated with a glutenfree diet for a period varying from 1-15 years (average 54 months). As during that period they were erroneously considered by themselves, their family and friends to suffer from CD, we coined the name "pseudo-CD" for this unnecessary clinical course. In a retrospective study we compared some of the main clinical and biochemical features of patients with CD (n=20), pseudo-CD (pCD) (n=15) and toddler's diarrhea (TD) (n=22) (10). The main results are summarized in Tables I-III.

TABLE I MAIN CLINICAL AND ANAMNESTIC FEATURES

	Chronical diarrhea	Ill temper	Failure to thrive	Abdominal distention	Positive family history
CD	12/19	10/15	19/19	14/16	0/20
	60%	67%	100%	87%	0%
pCD	4/15	6/15	5/15	5/15	11/15
	27%	40%	33%	33%	73%
TD	13/22	2/22	9/22	5/20	9/22
	59%	9%	41%	25%	9%

TABLE II LABORATORY INVESTIGATIONS

	Anaemia folic	Decreased acid	Decreased SeF	Abnormal xylose	AGA *	Abnormal fat excretion
CD	7/14	7/15	12/13	7/11	6/9	12/14
	50%	46%	86%	58%	66%	85%
pCD	0/7	1/14	5/14	2/14	2/7	1/4
	0%	7%	35%	14%	28%	25%
TD	0/20	2/18	8/18	2/18	4/9	1/9
	0%	11%	44%	11%	44%	11%

* Antigliadin antibodies: IgG + IgA > 0.7 O.D., investigation performed in the Laboratory of the Dep. of Gastroenterology, University of Leiden (A.S. Peña).

TABLE III DIAGNOSTIC DELAY

Mean age at:	Mean age at (months) start of symptoms	Mean age at (months) diagnosis
CD	8.7 (2-19)	66
pCD	17 (1-120)	90
TD	32.8 (1-168)	80

Despite the limitations of such a retrospective study the results suggest that there is a serious overlap in anamnestic, clinical and biochemical features between the three groups studied. Attention should be paid to the high incidence of a positive family history in the group of patients with "pseudo-CD". From these results one may conclude that the installation of a glutenfree diet without preceding examination of the small bowel mucosa may easily lead to an increase in diagnostic delay and unnecessary treatment with glutenfree diet with all its economic and psychosocial consequences.

THE BIOPSY CAPSULE

Although even today some reluctancy exists among physicians concerning peroral small intestinal biopsy, the first instrument, specifically designed to obtain samples of the small intestinal mucosa by peroral suction biopsy has been described already in the mid fifties (1,11,12). The capsule developed by Crosby and Kugler (13) providing more flexibility, has been used with success all over the world. Complications, including perforation, bleeding and dislodgement of the cap of the capsule, as well as modifications and adaptation to the use in pediatric patients, have been reported (14,15). A variety of different instruments has been presented in the last 20 years. Carey (16) developed a simplified biopsy capsule for obtaining multiple intestinal biopsy specimens in the office or at the bedside. The capsule described by Ament and Rubin (17) was a miniaturized version of the adult multi-purpose biopsy capsule that was described in 1959 (18). By reducing the diameter (3.5 mm versus 4.7 mm), the length (90 cm versus 120 cm) and increasing flexibility (radius of curvature 34 mm versus 40 mm), the capsule was easier to pass into the duodenum of children. A decrease in the diameter of the biopsy ports (2.0 mm versus 2.4 mm) allowed adequate size biopsies for diagnostic purposes with reduced risk of perforation. With this capsule in 69 of 102 patients, of which 27 weighed less than 10 kg, the biopsy procedure was successfully performed, resulting in 320 biopsies and a complication rate of less than 1%. Biopsies could be obtained in 78% of patients on the first attempt. However, using this technique it was necessary to remove the capsule from the patient in order to establish success of the procedure and/or the quality of the small intestinal mucosa sample taken. If unsuccessfull or if multiple biopsies were warranted for further diagnoses or different investigations, repeated intubation with positioning of the capsule had to be performed. Hydraulic biopsy capsules, described by several authors since the 1960-ies, have the advantage that multiple small bowel biopsies can be produces without removing the capsule from the intestinal tract. A diagram, describing the instrument's operation, is presented in figure I.

In 1-A a knuckle of mucosa is drawn into the biopsy capsule by applying negative pressure to the proximal end of the effluent channel. Fluid under pressure is pumped into the smaller effluent channel, closing the knife and excising the biopsy (B). The movement of the knife during closure opens a shunt which connects the effluent high pressure channel with the effluent low pressure channel. The specimen is now rapidly washed through the effluent channel to the exterior (C). After finishing this cycle the pressure is released and the spring-loaded knife springs open for the next biopsy procedure.

Flick and coworkers (23), using a hydraulic biopsy capsule, performed 160 biopsies in 8 patients during 11 intubations. No gross bleedings or perforations were seen. Some of the patients developed a post-biopsy syndrome consisting of abdominal

cramps and discomfort, following the procedure. Rubin and Dobbing performed 183 "hydraulic" biopsies in 118 intubations. They encountered no perforations, but 7 significant hemorrhages were seen, not requiring surgery or blood transfusion.
In an attempt to lower the threshold for small intestinal biopsy and to improve the efficiency of this diagnostic procedure, a new technique has been developed within the Departments of Pediatrics and Gastroenterology of the Academic Medical Center in Amsterdam.

FIGURE I

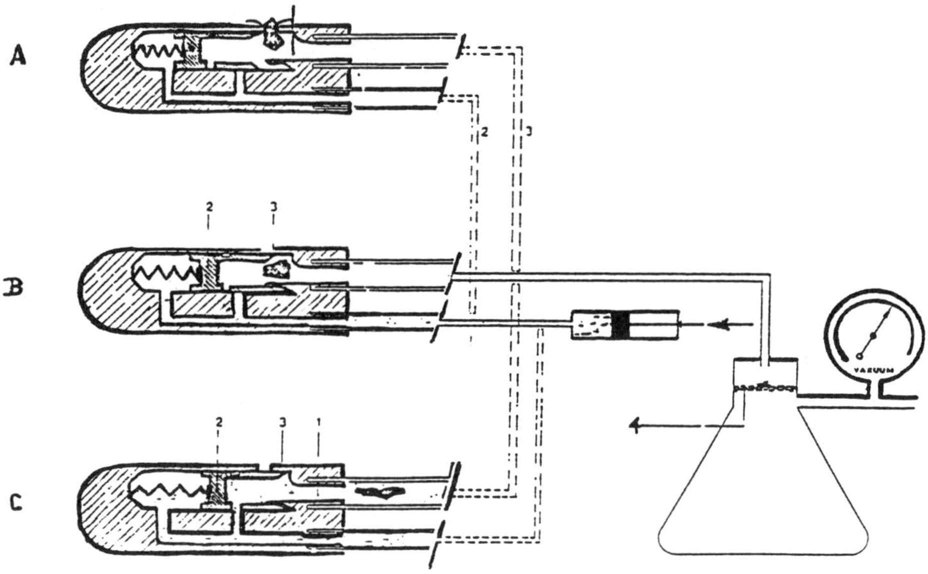

AMSTERDAM EXPERIENCE

A pediatric hydraulic biopsy capsule (Enraf Nonius, Delft, The Netherlands, length 21 mm, diameter 8 mm, biopsy port 2 mm) was connected to an hydraulic suction pump (Quinton Instruments Co., Seatle, Wash., USA) by two plastic tubes, one for hydraulic operation of the knife and the other for flushing the mucosa specimen. To allow quick passage to the duodenal jejunal flexure, a flexible iron guide wire was placed within one of the tubes before the capsule was advanced under fluoroscopic control. In this way more than 250 pediatric and 1200 adult patients have been investigated during the last 8 years. In less than 1% of the patients the procedure was not successfull in the first attempt. The only complication encountered was a severe bleeding in one adult patient that stopped spontaneously.
An average of 5 small intestinal biopsies per patient were available for investigations, including routine histology, immunofluorescence, electron microscopy and biochemical investigation of brush border enzymes. After adequate preparation of the patient including sedation in smaller pediatric patients this procedure took ± 15 minutes per patient and was easily performed on an outpatient basis. Recently it has been suggested that endoscopes capable of obtaining jumbo biopsies (8 mm open span)

provide tissue that is comparable in size to suction biopsies.
Especially in pediatric patients we would like to follow recommendations of the working group of ESPGAN (6), that small intestinal mucosal biopsies should always be taken with a biopsy capsule rather than through the endoscope to ensure diagnostically adequate specimens that may be orientated correctly for histological sections.

CONCLUSIONS

For the diagnosis of CD investigation of the small intestinal mucosa is mandatory. Installation of a glutenfree diet without preceding investigation of the small intestinal mucosa can result in diagnostic delay and unnecessary treatment with severe financial and psychosocial implications. Patients, their parents and some physicians consider small bowel biopsies still as a very unpleasant invasive diagnostic technique. This has resulted in reluctancy to apply the technique, even when indicated. With the use of the hydraulic pediatric capsules, an efficient, save and elegant diagnostic technique has become available, for both pediatric and adult patients, that will contribute to the diagnosis of CD.

REFERENCES

1 Royer M. Biopsia duodenal por aspiraci6n bajo control radiosc6pico. Prensa Med Argent 1955;42:2515.
2 Trier JS. Diagnostic value of peroral biopsy of the proximal small intestine. New Engl J Med 1971;285:1470.
3 Meuwisse GW. Diagnostic criteria in coeliac disease. Acta Paed Scand 1970;59:461.
4 Visakorpi JK. Definition of coeliac disease in children. In: Hekkens WTJM and Pena AS (eds.), Coeliac diseases. Proceeding of the Second International Coeliac Symposium, Noordwijkerhout, Stenfert Kroese 1974;10-6.
5 McNeish AS. Re-evaluation of diagnostic criteria for coeliac disease. Arch Dis Childh 1979;54:783.
6 Walker-Smith JA. Revised criteria for diagnosis of coeliac disease. Report of the Working Group of the European Society of Paediatric Gastroenterology and Nutrition. Arch Dis Childh 1990;65:909.
7 Anderson CM. Coeliac disease: some still controversial aspects. Arch Dis Childh 1972;47:292.
8 Schubert WK. Treatment, but with inadequate diagnosis? Pediatrics 1978;61:930.
9 Lloyd-Still JD. Where have all the celiacs gone? Pediatrics 1978;61:929.
10 Walker-Smith JA. Toddler's diarrhea. Arch Dis Childh 1980;55:329.
11 Shiner M. Duodenal biopsy. Lancet 1956;I:17.
12 Shiner M. Jejunal biopsy tube. Lancet 1956;I:85.
13 Crosby WH. Intraluminal biopsy of the small intestine. The intestinal biopsy capsule. Am J Digest Dis 1957;2:236.
14 Read AE. An improvement to the Crosby peroral intestinal biopsy capsule. Lancet 1962;I:894.
15 Kilby A. Paediatric small intestinal biopsy capsule with two ports. Gut 1976;17:158.
16 Carey JB. A simplified gastrointestinal biopsy capsule. Gastroent 1964;46:550.
17 Ament ME. An infant multipurpose biopsy tube. Gastroent 1973;65:205.
18 Brandborg LL. A multipurpose instrument for suction biopsy of the esophagus, stomach, small bowel and colon. Gastroent 1959;37:1.
19 Henning N. An instrument for mucosal biopsy from small and large intestine. German Med Month 1960;5:13.
20 Baker SJ. Multi-retrieving small intestinal biopsy tube. Lancet 1960;II:686.
21 Ross JR. Small intestinal biopsy capsule utilizing hydrostatic and suction principles. Gastroent 1961;40:113.
22 Lehmann KE. An instrument for multiple transoral biopsies of the gastro-intestinal tract. Acta Med Scand 1961;169:205.

23 Flick AL. A peroral hydraulic biopsy tube for multiple sampling at any level of the gastrointestinal tract. Gastroent 1961;40:120.
24 Bolt R. A simplified multiple-retrieving small bowel biopsy tube. Am J Dig Dis 1962;7:773.
25 Rubin CE. Peroral biopsy of the small intestine. A review of its diagnostic usefulness. Gastroent 1965;49:676.
26 Riddell RH. Small intestinal biopsy: who, how, what are the findings? In: Barkin JS, Rogers (AI (eds.), Different decisions in digestive diseases. Year Book Medical Publishers Inc., Chicago, 1989;326.

HIGH INCIDENCE OF ATYPICAL FORMS OF COELIAC DISEASE IN A PEDIATRIC CASE STUDY.

M. Castro, *G. Castellucci, B. Papadatou, M. Gambarara, V. Lucidi, F. Ferretti, S. Bella, A.M. Colombo. Ospedale Bambino Gesù, divisione di Gastroenterologia, Roma. *Clinica pediatrica Università di Perugia.

INTRODUCTION

In the last ten years, better knowledge of coeliac disease (CD), has permitted the identification, not only of the typical forms of the disease characterized by gastrointestinal symptoms, but the identification of atypical forms, characterized by the absence of diarrhea and the presence, sometimes, of symptoms not referring to a gastrointestinal pathology. In the beginning such atypical forms were considered rather rare and more frequent in older children but we are becoming more and more convinced that there is an increase of the number of such atypical diagnostic forms. This is due above all, either to the greater sensibilization of both pediatric gastroenterologists and pediatricians, or the use of new screening tests for CD like the antigliadin antibodies, that allow us to choose the subjects to present for biopsy. In the last 12 years, at our center in Rome, 352 cases of CD, aged 8 months to 16 years, have been diagnosed by jejunal biopsy. Of these 279 patients, that is 79%, were affected by a typical form, and 73 patients, that is 21%, presented an atypical clinical picture, without the classic symptoms of CD, at the moment of the diagnosis. The percentage of atypical forms diagnosed by our center six years ago was 11% and that percentage increased in the last years to 21%. Half of the atypical forms had had an early beginning within the first 3 years of life, while the other half had a retarded beginning after the first three years (Table I).

TABLE I DISTRIBUTION OF THE CLINICAL PICTURE IN 352 COELIAC CHILDREN

Total coeliacs (352 p.) →	Typical forms: 79% (279 p.) →	< 3 yrs: 202 (57%)
		> 3 yrs: 77 (22%)
	Atypical forms: 21% (73 p.) →	< 3 yrs: 37 (10.5%)
		> 3 yrs: 36 (10.5%)

There was no difference between the two groups (typical and atypical) as far as concerns the duration of breast-feeding, while the mean age in which gluten was introduced into the diet was 4 months for the patients with typical form and 6 months for the children with atypical one. There was a different latency between the two groups. In the typical forms the mean latency was 4.4 months while in the atypical ones the mean latency reaches approximatly 15 months, even if we were not

M. L. Mearin and C. J. J. Mulder (eds.), Coeliac Disease, 165–168.

able to determine the exact pointed time of onset in all patients because the symptoms appeared very gradually in some of them. We have divided the whole group of coeliac patients into two groups according to age (above and below 3 years of age). In the younger group of coeliac patients (239 children), atypical forms resulted in 37 patients, that is 15%, while in the older children (113 patients) the incidence of atypical forms was higher equal to 32%; thus the percentage of atypical forms is much higher in older coeliac patients and reaches 1/3 of the total older coeliac children (Table II).

TABLE II DISTRIBUTION OF THE CLINICAL PICTURE ACCORDING TO THE AGE OF PRESENTATION

Total coeliacs (352 p.) →	age < 3 yrs 239 p. (68%) →	typical forms : 202 (85%) atypical forms: 37 (15%)
Total coeliacs (352 p.) →	age > 3 yrs 113 p. (32%) →	typical forms : 77 (68%) atypical forms: 36 (32%)

Table III shows the symptoms and signs, presented by the patients affected by atypical forms of CD. The most frequently observed symptom was delayed weight growth (44% of the patients), while stunted growth was found in 27% of the patients especially in those over three years of age. Anorexia was present in 34% of the patients, and vomiting in 27%. The patient with hypocalcemia was affected by Down's syndrome and was treated for rickets before the diagnosis of CD was made. The total of the percentages exceeds 100% because more than one symptom was present in the same patient.

TABLE III ATYPICAL FORMS OF CD: SYMPTOMS AND SIGNS

Weight < 3d percentile	32 (44%)
Anorexia	25 (34%)
Height < 3d percentile	20 (27%)
Vomiting	20 (27%)
Height and weight < 3d percentile	13 (18%)
Meteorism	10 (14%)
Constipation	10 (14%)
Recurrent abdominal pain	5 (7%)
Anaemia	3 (4%)
Oedemas	2 (3%)
Hypocalcemia	1 (1%)

Table IV shows the symptoms present in our patients according to age. Vomiting was present only in the younger group, while isolated stunted growth was more frequently present in the older group (14 versus 3%). Recurrent abdominal pain was more frequent in younger patients. Anemia as a singular symptom and hypocalcemia were present in older patients. It must be pointed out that about 1/3 of the atypical coeliac patients over 3 years of age showed a positive history of diarrhea in early age, and in most cases they were treated with gluten-free diet for a few months without specific investigation. Such a behaviour may have altered the natural history of the disease, therefore it would be more correct to call these cases "pseudo-atypical" ones.

The retrospective analysis of our case studies permit us to make several considerations:

- atypical forms of CD represent more than 20% of all diagnosis;
- there are precocious and delated atypical forms;
- the incidence of the delated atypical forms is higher than the incidence of the precocious ones;
- there is a different distribution of symptoms according to age;
- it is probable (even in our days) that the atypical forms of CD are not diagnosed in alle cases and consequently the true incidence of CD is underestimated.

TABLE IV ATYPICAL FORMS OF CD: SYMPTOMS AND SIGNS

	Coeliac p.<3 yrs (37 p.)	Coeliac p.>3 yrs (36 p.)
Vomiting	20 (54%)	- -
Anorexia	16 (43%)	8 (22%)
Weight < 3d percentile	16 (43%)	4 (11%)
Weight and height < 3d percentile	8 (22%)	10 (28%)
Constipation	7 (19%)	3 (8%)
Meteorism	5 (14%)	5 (14%)
R.A.P.	2 (5%)	4 (11%)
Oedemas	2 (5%)	- -
Height < 3d percentile	1 (3%)	5 (14%)
Anaemia	- -	3 (8%)
Hypocalcemia	- -	1 (3%)

REFERENCES

1 Anderson CM, Gracey M, Burke V. Coeliac disease. Some still controversial aspects. Arch Dis Child 1972;47:292.

2 Banchini G, De Angelis GL, Gregori G, Zanacca C, Volta C, Bernasoni S, Giovanelli C. La bassa statura come manifestazione principale della malattia celiaca. Valutazione auxologica

prima e dopo dieta senza glutine. Riv Ital Ped 1984;10:229.
3 Barry RE, Baker P, Read AE. Coeliac disease. The clinical presentation. Clin Gastroenterol 1974;3:55.
4 Castro M, Lucidi V, Papadatou B. La malattia celiaca: considerazioni a proposito di 18 pazienti di età superiore a 3 anni. Rass Ital Chir Ped Vol XXIV 1982;4 (suppl).
5 Groll a, Candy DCA, Preece MA, Tanner JM, Harris JT. Short stature as the primary manifestation of coelaic disease. Lancet II 1980;1097.
6 Labenthal E, Branski D. Childhood coeliac disease a reappriasal. J Pediatr 1981;98:681.
7 Lloyd-Still JD. Where have all the coeliacs gone? Pediatrics 1978;61:929.
8 Rossi E. Monosymptomatic forms of coeliac disease. Eur J Pediatr 1982;138:4.

COELIAC DISEASE IN THE NETHERLANDS.

T.L.T.A. Jansen, C.G.J. Wagenaar, C.J.J. Mulder. Dep. Hepatogastroenterology, Rijnstate Hospital, Dutch Coeliac Society, P.O. BOX 9555, 6800 TA Arnhem, The Netherlands.

Epidemiologic studies in the past have demonstrated internationally varying prevalence of coeliac disease (CD). To update Dutch data we analyzed the records of members of the Dutch Coeliac Society. At January 1st 1990 1705 unselected members were counted. Twelve hundred thirtythree were at least single-biopsy confirmed coeliacs. Since 1980 1110 new patients have been registered, of which 783 (=70½%) were biopsy-proven. CD became manifest most frequently in the first decade (33%) and in the fourth and fifth decades (35%) of life. Most cases, however, were diagnosed in adults: 62%. An interesting variation was observed in the estimate of prevalence rates (per 100.000 inhabitants) in different geographical areas. The overall prevalence rate in the Netherlands was 10.8; the lowest prevalence rate was found in Flevoland (5.9), the highest in Utrecht (17.7). These rates were less in the greater cities (>100.000 inhabitants), than in a selected group of welfaring, smaller cities (<60.00 inhabitants): respectively (mean+SD) 11.7+4.9 vs 20.5+13.7; $p<0.05$. Incidence rates (per 100.000 inhabitants/yr) increased from 0.13 in 1975, 0.22 in 1980, 0.45 in 1985 to 0.89 in 1989. This increase in coeliac diagnoses outranged the mean increase of the Dutch population over the last decade (+0.5%/yr). We conclude that the number of known coeliacs is low in comparison to neighbouring countries, but in the Netherlands it increases enormously during the last decade. Incidence rates and geographically-varying prevalence rates suggest that other than population factors are causative. To substantiate causes of this increase further analysis is warranted. We hypothesize that medical inattention, in part (still) might explain the low Dutch overall prevalence, as well as the low prevalence in several geographical areas.

INTRODUCTION

Since the first classical description by Samuel Gee in 1888, CD has been recognized by clinicians for one century (1). It was not untill the early fourties that Dicke in collaboration with Weyers and Van de Kamer discovered the crucial role of gluten in the pathogenesis of the steatorrhoea (2,3). A few years later, the introduction of the small-intestinal biopsy technique allowed the pathological recognition of the characteristic lesion in the jenunal mucosa of CD (4). The Dutch Coeliac Disease Society was conceived at the end of the 2nd International Conference on CD (5), held in Noordwijkerhout on September 21st 1974 by a group of patients with collaboration of some Board Members of the Coeliac Society of the United Kingdom. Little is known about CD in The Netherlands on national level (6). We tried to gather some data by examining the CD society membership records; such an analysis has also been made in Great Britain and New Zealand (7,8). In this study we report the analysis of the membership records of the Dutch Coeliac Society at January 1st 1990. The records of Coeliac Society memberships are at this moment the

M. L. Mearin and C. J. J. Mulder (eds.), Coeliac Disease, 169–179.

best source on CD, and give in all probability only a slight underestimate of the true prevalence of CD (5), because CD patients get (non)financial advantages by their membership.

MATERIALS AND METHODS

Analysis of the membership records:
at January 1st, the records of 1705 members of the Dutch Coeliac Society were analysed. Of these 1233 were biopsy-proven and 154 not biopsy-proven coeliacs (N=1387). These computer data gave information on sex, date of birth, year of diagnosis, year of registration, hospital of diagnosis and availability of jejunal biopsy. Names were for ethical reasons not available for the investigators. Epidemiological data of the general population were obtained from the Central Bureau for Statistics (CBS) (9).

Statistical analysis:
statistical analysis was performed using Student's t-test. To evaluate the difference between groups, data of these groups were compared with each other by using unpaired Student's t-test. Significance was accepted at the 0.05 level of probability (two-sided).

Data report:
number of inhabitants per region or city is given as published by CBS (9). Prevalence and incidence rates are demonstrated per 100.000 inhabitants. Biopsy-rates are expressed in percentage. All results are expressed as mean values ± standard deviation (SD), unless indicated otherwise.

RESULTS

Prevalence rate:
the prevalence rates of coeliacs per province are presented in table I. From the records 1204 (98%) of 1233 biopsy-proven coeliacs could be traced to a province. The mean provincial prevalence rate (per 100.000 inhabitants) was 7.9 ± 2.2, with 95% lower and upper confidence limits of 6.6 and 9.3 respectively.
An extreme low, even below the lower 95% confidence levels, prevalence rate was observed in Groningen 6.1, Flevoland 5.4 and Zeeland 5.9. Beyond the upper 95% confidence limits, high prevalence rates were observed in Gelderland 9.6 and Utrecht 13.4. Other provincial prevalence rates were not surprisingly different from the mean.
The prevalence rates of CD in the great cities, i.e. more than 100.000 inhabitants, are presented in table II. In these 16 cities 25% (3.760.235 of 14.805.240 inhabitants) of the general Dutch population lived; of them 247 (21%) of all 1204 biopsy-proven coeliac patients lived: meaning a prevalence rate of 6.6 per 100.000 inhabitants.
The mean urban prevalence rate (per 100.000 inhabitants) was 7.7±2.8, with 95% lower and upper confidence limits of 6.2 and 9.2 respectively. An extreme low, even

below the lower 95% confidence limits, prevalence rate was observed in Amsterdam 5.2, Apeldoorn 4.8, Haarlem 5.4, and Rotterdam 3.1. High prevalence rates, even beyond the upper 95% confidence limits, were observed in Leiden 13.7, Nijmegen 11.7 and Utrecht 11.7. Other urban prevalence rates were not surprisingly different from the mean urban prevalence rate.

TABLE I REGIONAL PREVALENCE RATES (PER 100.000 INHABITANTS) OF 1204 BIOPSY-PROVENCOELIAC PATIENTS, KNOWN TO THE DUTCH COELIAC SOCIETY.

Province	Inhabitants (N)	Coeliacs (N)	Prevalence (N/10.5)	Biopsy (%) proven	not-proven
Drenthe	439.066	33	7.5	94	6
Friesland	599.190	56	9.3	85	15
Gelderland	1.794.678	173	9.6	93	7
Groningen	555.200	34	6.1	92	8
Limburg	1.099.622	75	6.8	88	12
Noord-Brabant	2.172.604	158	7.3	88	12
Noord-Holland	2.365.160	189	8.0	84	16
Overijssel	1.014.949	87	8.6	88	12
Flevoland	202.678	11	5.4	92	8
Utrecht	1.004.632	135	13.4	97	3
Zeeland	355.585	21	5.9	78	22
Zuid-Holland	3.200.408	232	7.2	88	12
Mean			7.9		
± S.D.			2.2		
95% Conf. limits			6.6-9.3		
Total	14.805.240	1204			

Numbers are demonstrated from the 12 Dutch provinces, with rates of biopsyproven celiac diagnoses. Data from the general population are from January 1 st 1989 as published by CBS.

The prevalence rates of CD in a selected group of small cities, i.e. with less than 60.000 inhabitants, are presented in table III. In the upper part **A**, a selected group of 10 welfaring cities are tabled. Only 274.635 (1.9%) people lived in these cities. The mean prevalence of CD was surprisingly high: 18.3±13.9, and higher than the mean prevalence rate in the greater cities, P=0.006. In the lower part **B**, an aselected group of small cities was matched to **A**. In these 401.579 (2.7%) people were living. The mean prevalence of CD in group **B** cities was surprisingly low: 1.9±3.0. This was significantly lower than the mean prevalence rate in the selected group of cities, P=0.002, and lower than the mean prevalence rate in the greater cities, P=0.001.

Incidence rate:
the incidence rates (per 100.000 inhabitants) of CD are demonstrated in figure 1 per year (1975 - 1989). Comparing the curve of incidence rates with the curve of population increase a significant difference with $P<0.05$ is revealed. Since 1975 the general population has increased with $+0.7\pm0.24$ % per year. Incidence of CD increased every year, from +0.13 patients/10.5 inhabitants in 1975 to +0.89 patients/10.5 inhabitants in 1989. In fact, incidence grew quite suddenly from 1981.

TABLE II URBAN PREVALANCE RATES (PER 100.000 INHABITANTS) OF COELIAC PATIENTS, KNOWN TO THE DUTCH COELIAC SOCIETY

Cities	Inhabitants (N)	Coeliacs (N)	Prevalence (N/10.5 inh.)	Biopsy (%) proven	not-proven
Amsterdam	694.680	36	5.2	92	8
Apeldoorn	147.270	7	4.8	100	0
Arnhem	128.946	9	7.0	100	0
Breda	121.362	8	6.6	73	27
Den Haag	443.845	33	7.4	87	13
Dordrecht	108.519	9	8.3	90	10
Eindhoven	190.736	17	8.9	89	11
Enschede	145.223	9	6.2	90	10
Groningen	167.788	12	7.2	92	8
Haarlem	149.198	8	5.4	80	20
Leiden	109.254	15	13.7	88	12
Maastricht	116.380	10	8.6	83	17
Nijmegen	145.405	17	11.7	94	6
Rotterdam	576.232	18	3.1	78	22
Tilburg	155.110	12	7.7	80	20
Utrecht	230.634	27	11.7	100	0
Mean	221.190		7.7		
± S.D.			2.8		
95% Conf. limits			6.2-9.2		
Total	3.760.235	247			

Numbers are demonstrated from the 17 greatest (>100.000 inh.) Dutch cities, with rates of biopsy proven coeliac diagnoses.

Age of coeliac patients:
the age of all biopsy-proven coeliacs registered at the Dutch Coeliac Society is demonstrated in figure 2. Interestingly only 31% of the 1233 biopsy-proven coeliacs was 0 - 20 of which 14% was 0 - 10 years of age, and 45% was 35 - 65 years of age. More than 75% of coeliac patients were either between 0 and 20, or between 35 and 65 year. Only 11% of the 1233 biopsy-proven coeliacs was 20 -35 years of age; and 12.5% of the 1233 biopsy-proven coeliacs was beyond 65 years of age.

The age of patients at the time of diagnosis is showed in figure 3. The age at time of diagnosis was available in 1216 (98.6%) of the 1233 biopsy-proven-coeliac membership records. In 33% of the patients CD had been diagnosed at an age of less than 10 years. In this age-group the female/male ratio was 1.75 (N=380). Only 4.1 % of patients was diagnosed in the second decade of life. After the second decade of life in 62% of patients CD had been diagnosed. In 9.3% of patients CD had been diagnosed at 60 years of age or beyond. In this age-group the female/male ratio was 1.76 (N=94).

FIGURE I

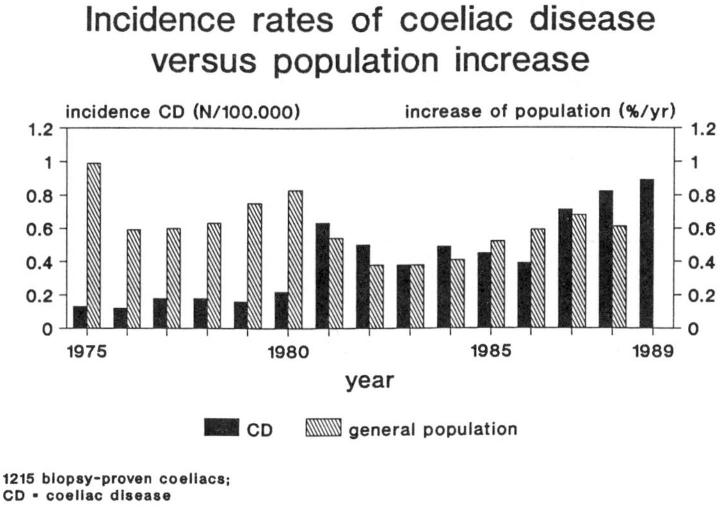

FIGURE II

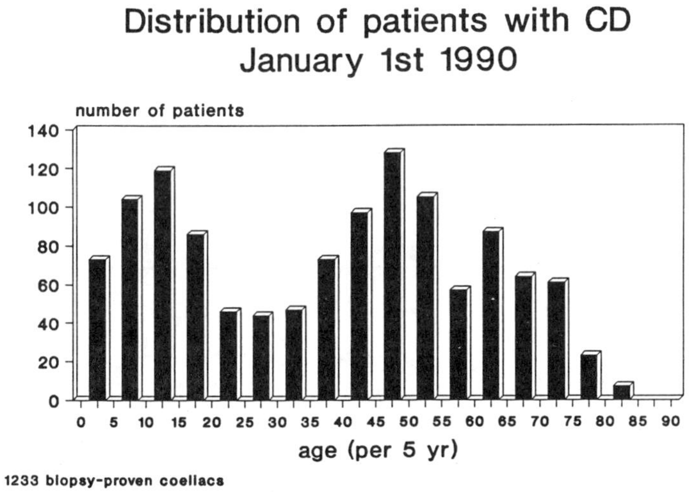

TABLE III-A URBAN PREVALANCE RATES (PER 100.000 INHABITANTS) OF COELIAC PATIETNS, KNOWN TO THE DUTCH COELIAC SOCIETY

Cities	Inhabitants (N)	Coeliacs (N)	Prevalence ($N/10^5$ inh.)	Biopsy (%) proven	not prove
Assen	49.398	5	10.1	83	17
Blaricum	10.775	6	55.7	100	0
Bloemendaal	17.412	1	5.7	33	67
Bussum	31.988	6	18.8	86	14
Goes	31.815	6	18.9	100	0
Haren	18.228	2	11.0	67	33
Laren	11.643	2	17.2	100	0
Roosendaal	59.237	6	10.1	100	0
Oegstgeest	18.167	3	16.5	75	25
Wassenaar	25.972	5	19.3	100	0
Mean	30.474	51	18.3		
± S.D.			13.9		
95% Conf. limits			8.4-28.3		
Total	274.635				

TABLE III-B

Almelo	62.008	6	9.7	75	25
Delfzijl	23.472	1	4.3		
Doesburg	10.578	0	0		
Doetinchem	41.260	0	0		
Helmond	66.791	1	1.5		
Hulst	18.575	0	0		
Lelystad	58.125	1	1.7		
Smallingerland	50.434	0	0		
Urk	12.728	0	0		
Velsen	57.608	1	1.7		
Mean	29.103	7	1.9		
± S.D.	18.082		3.0		
95% Conf. limits			-0.3-4.1		
Total	401.579				

Numbers are demonstrated in A from some (<60.000 inh.) Dutch cities, and in B from an aselected group of small cities; rates are shown from percentage in which biopsy-proof was obtained to diagnosis.

From 1955 to 1989 the age at time of diagnosis was increasing, as demonstrated in table IV. In blocks of 5 year the mean age at time of diagnosis is demonstrated from 1257 patients, of which 1233 patients were biopsy-proven. The mean age increased from 19.5±16.3 in 1955-1959 (N=8) to 33.2±24.6 yr in 1985-1989 (N=396).

FIGURE III

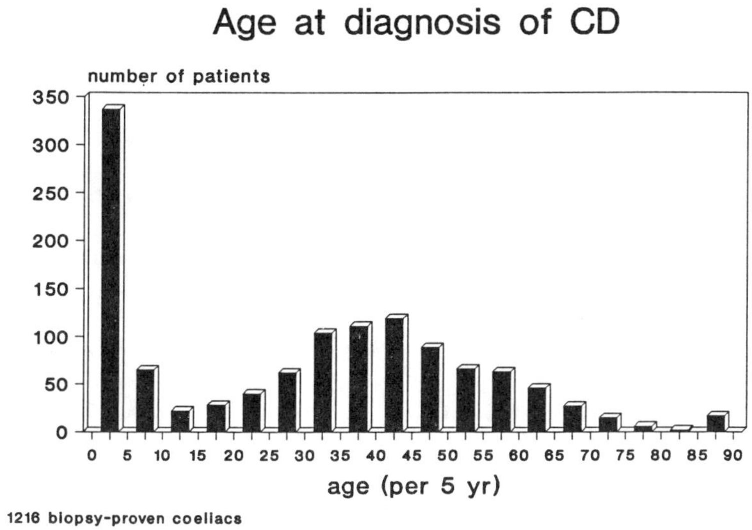

TABLE IV MAEN AGE AT DIAGNOSIS OF COELIAC DISEASE PER 5 YEARS IN N=1257, OFWHICH 1233 BIOPSY-PROVEN COELIACS

	mean age (yr)	SD (yr)	min (yr)	max (yr)	N
1955 - 1959	19.5	16.3	1	41	8
1960 - 1964	31.2	18.1	0	57	21
1965 - 1969	26.2	18.9	1	56	44
1970 - 1974	28.1	20.7	1	71	140
1975 - 1979	25.6	21.9	0	77	249
1980 - 1984	28.9	21.9	0	85	399
1985 - 1989	33.2	24.6	0	89	396
Total					1257

Sex-rate: both the age of patients at the time of diagnosis and sex-rate are demonstrated in table V. The sex was available in 1182 of 1216 cases of which age at time of diagnosis was known. CD was diagnosed more often in females than in males: overall female/male rate 2.02 (N=1182). High sex-rates were observed in several age groups: (female/male-rate) 2.9 at 21 - 35 yr and 6.0 beyond 86 yr.

Biopsy-rate: the numbers of cases at which biopsy was taken to prove villous atrophy, are demonstrated in the tables I, II and III. The mean percentage of biopsy-proven cases was 88.9±5.1% in the 12 Dutch provinces, table I. High biopsy-rates, even beyond the 95% confidence limits, were observed in Drenthe 94%, Gelderland 93% and Utrecht 97%. Low biopsyrates, below the 95% confidence limits, were observed in Noord-Holland 84% and Zeeland 78%. The mean percentage of biopsy-proven cases was 88.5±8.1% in the 16 greatest Dutch cities, table II. High biopsy-rates, even beyond the 95% confidence limits, were observed in Apeldoorn 100%, Arnhem 100%, Nijmegen 94% and Utrecht 100%. Low biopsyrates, below the 95% confidence limits, were observed in Breda 73%, Haarlem 80% and Maastricht 83%. Biopsy-rates in the 16 greates cities were not significantly different from rates in the 12 Dutch provinces. The mean percentage of biopsy-proven cases was 84.4±21.7% in a selected group of 10 small Dutch cities, table III **A**. High biopsy-rates, even beyond the 95% confidence limits, were observed in Blaricum 100%, Goes 100%, Laren 100%, Roosendaal 100% and Wassenaar 100%. Low biopsy-rates, even below the 95% confidence limits, were observed in Bloemendaal 33% and Haren 67%. Biopsy-rates in the 10 small cities were not significantly different from rates in the 12 Dutch provinces or from the 16 greatest cities.

TABLE V AGE AT DIAGNOSIS OF COELIAC DISEASE AND SEX-RATES PER 5 YEARS IN 1182 BIOPSY-PROVEN COELIACS

	Male (N)	Female (N)	Female/male-rate
0 - 5	107	211	1.97
6 - 10	31	31	1.00
11 - 15	8	11	1.38
16 - 20	9	14	1.56
21 - 25	10	36	3.60
26 - 30	18	56	3.11
31 - 35	31	78	2.52
36 - 40	38	72	1.89
41 - 45	43	80	1.86
46 - 50	21	55	2.62
51 - 55	24	41	1.71
56 - 60	17	46	2.71
61 - 65	18	20	1.11
66 - 70	8	17	2.13
71 - 75	3	9	3.00
76 - 80	1	1	1.00
81 - 85	2	1	0.50
86 - 90	2	12	6.00
Total	391	791	2.02

Dermatitis Herpetiformis: figure 4 demonstrates the age-plot of 29 (2.1% of all 1387 coeliacs) coeliac patients of which the records consist information on having dermatitis herpetiformis. The peak age conforms to the second peak age in figure 3.

FIGURE IV

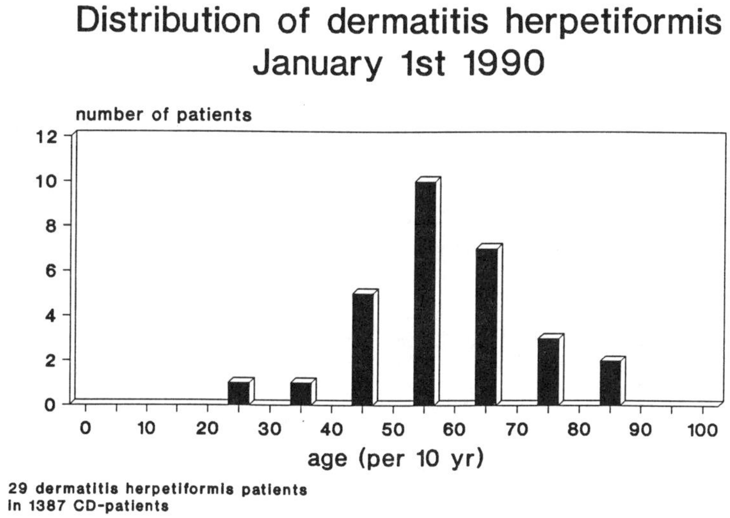

DISCUSSION

In the present study we have examined the epidemiology of biopsy-proven CD, as it is presented to the Dutch Coeliac Society. It is based on the principle that most coeliacs have inscribed as members of this Society, as membership gives certain advantages. Members are informed about novelties on their disease and diet, as well as about Society-events. More directly, members can buy gluten-free products at discount prices. The present study showed interesting data on prevalence of CD. A three-fold variation in the estimate of prevalence rates in different geographical areas was observed. In different geographical areas a two- to three-fold variation has been described before (6,7,8). The overall prevalence rate in The Netherlands was 11 per 100.000 inhabitants; still low when compared to the English prevalence estimate (in 1980) of 27 per 100.000 inhabitants, but doubling since 1983 (6). The prevalence rates obtained in this survey are probably still a slight underestimate of the true prevalence of CD in The Netherlands. Surprising high prevalence rates (18.3± 13.9/10.5 inhabitants) were obtained from a selected group of welfaring small cities. A group of cities, equal in size, was aselectively matched to these welfaring small cities. Prevalence of CD in this matched group of cities (1.9±3.0/10.5 inhabitants) was significantly lower. Prevalence of CD in the group of great cities (7.7±2.8/10.5 inhabitants) was significantly lower from prevalence in the welfaring small cities, as well. These data suggest that prosperity is positively associated to higher prevalence rates of recognized CD. The identity of this association remains unclear, and warrants further investigation, but it might be explained by second opinions outside the local region. Very few patients, only 4%, were diagnosed in the second decade. This finding is similar to other epidemiological studies (7,8). In contrast to others, we found that only 1.7% of patients were diagnosed in the eighth decade. Interestingly, however, after the 85th year 17 (1.4%) new patients were diagnosed. This might be a group that is first recognized during investigation and treatment of other more serious conditions, some of which are associated with CD (10,11). Observing the age-plots of CD-patients, an important number of patients is missing from 15 till 45 years. These missing patients might be explained by underdiagnosis during the sixties and seventies. Another interesting phenomenon is the rising mean age at time of diagnosis that we found comparing mean ages at time of diagnosis from before 1960 with mean ages from after 1980. These increasing mean ages, together with increasing maximum ages at time of diagnosis support the idea of underdiagnosis. Moreover rising maximum ages support the hypothesis that a group of patients is only first recognized during investigation and treatment of other more serious conditions, some of which are associated with CD.

TABLE VI INCIDENCE RATES (PER 100.000 INHABITANTS) OF COELIAC PATIENTS, KNOWN TO THE DUTCH COELIAC SOCIETY; WITH RATES OF BIOPSY-PROVEN COELIACS

Year	Inhabitants	Increase	Coeliacs			
		Prevalence	Increase	Increase	Incidence	
	(N)	(%/yr)	(N)	(N)	(%)	(N/10)
1975	13.599.092	0.99	311	18	5.8	0.13
1976	13.733.578	0.59	329	17	5.2	0.12
1977	13.814.495	0.60	346	25	7.2	0.18
1978	13.897.874	0.63	371	25	6.7	0.18
1979	13.985.526	0.75	396	23	5.8	0.16
1980	14.091.014	0.83	419	31	7.4	0.22
1981	14.208.586	0.54	450	89	19.8	0.63
1982	14.285.829	0.38	539	72	13.4	0.50
1983	14.339.551	0.38	611	54	8.8	0.38
1984	14.394.589	0.41	665	71	10.7	0.49
1985	14.453.833	0.52	736	65	8.8	0.45
1986	14.529.430	0.59	801	57	7.1	0.39
1987	14.615.125	0.68	858	104	12.1	0.71
1988	14.714.948	0.61	962	121	12.6	0.82
1989	14.805.240		1083	132	12.2	0.89
Mean		0.61				
± S.D.		0.1				
Total			1215			

This study suggests that prevalence is correlated to prosperity. Symptoms are initially non-specific, patients drift into ill-health and may be wrongly diagnosed initially. Prosperity might be a clue for second opinions and reconsidering patient-histories. The records of the Dutch Coeliac Society are the only national source of information on CD. Increasing incidence rates, especially after 1983, possibly a catch up manoevre from underdiagnosis in the past, suggest that greater awareness for CD by clinicians is going on. Case reports might sensitize clinicians so that they become aware of minor symptoms, and must realize that the so-called typical picture of CD, i.e. as diarrhoeal illness with frequent, foul-smelling, bulky stools and weight loss, only occurs in a minority of CD patients. On many occasions the clinical presentation is monosymptomatic, e.g. anaemia, osteoporosis, short stature and infertility (12-14). Enhanced awareness of the protean presentation might be helpfull.

FIGURE V

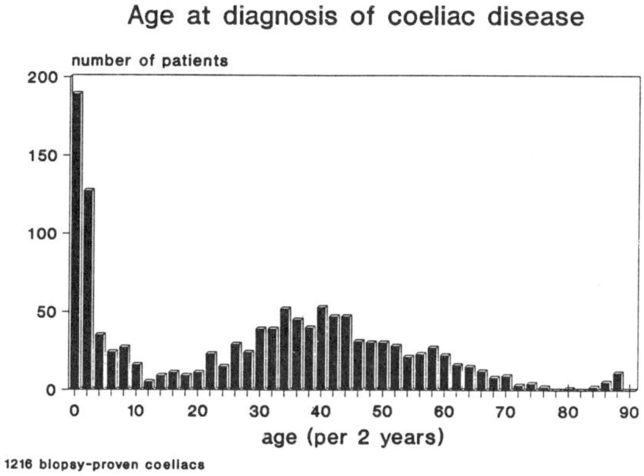

REFERENCES

1 Gee S. On the coeliac affection. St Bart's Hosp Rep 1888;24:17-20.
2 Dicke WK. Coeliac disease: investigation of the harmfull effects of certain types of cereal on patients with coeliac disease. M.D. thesis, University of Utrecht May 30th, 1950.
3 Dicke WK, Weyers HA, Van de Kamer JH. Coeliac Disease II: The presence in wheat of a factor having a deleterious effect in cases of coeliac disease. Acta Pediatr. 1953;42:43-52.
4 Doniach I, Shiner M. Duodenal and jejunal biopsies II. Histology Gastroenterology 1957;33:71-86.
5 Hekkens WTJM, Pena AS. eds. Proceedings of the 2nd International Symposium on Coeliac Disease. Leiden: Stenfert Kroese 1974.
6 Biemond I, Pena AS, Groenland F, Mulder CJJ, Tijtgat GNJ. Coeliac disease in The Netherlands. Neth J Med 1987;31:263-8.
7 McConnell RB. Membership of the Coeliac Society of the United Kingdom. In McConnell R.B. ed. The genetics of coeliac disease. Liverpool: MTP Press 1979:65-9.
8 Carrington JM. Coeliac disease: an analysis of Coeliac Society membership records. NZ Med J 1986;99:279-81.
9 Population of the municipalities of The Netherlands at Januari 1st 198). The Hague: SDU/publishers. Netherlands central bureau of statistics.
10 Logan RFA, Rifkind EA, Turner ID, and Ferguson A. Mortality in celiac disease. Gastroenterology 1989;97:265-71.
11 Mulder CJJ, Tytgat GNJ. Coeliac disease and related disorders. Neth J Med 1987;31:286-99.
12 Rossi E. Monosymptomatic forms of celiac disease. Eur J Pediatr 1982;138:4-5.
13 Editorial. Infertility in coeliac disease. Lancet 1983;1:453-4.
14 Depla ACTM, Bartelsman JFWM, Mulder CJJ, Tytgat GNJ. Anemia: monosymptomatic coeliac disease. Hepatogastroenterology 1990;37:90-91

IGA RETICULIN ANTIBODY BINDING TO HUMAN JEJUNUM IN SERA OF CHILDREN WITH COELIAC DISEASE: THE POSSIBLE AUTOANTIBODY OF GLUTEN SENSITIVE ENTEROPATHY

S. Karpati, A. Bürgin-Wolff, M. Meurer, Th. Krieg. Heim Pal Hospital for Children, Budapest, Hungary. Dermatological Clinic, Ludwig-Maximilians University, Munich, FRG. Dep. of Microbiology and Immunology, University Children's Hospital, Basel, Switzerland.

We recently described IgA antibody in sera of patients with dermatitis herpetiformis (DH) binding to human small bowel tissue in a similar way to tissue bound IgA in the jejunum of DH and coeliac disease (CD) patients (1-3). The purpose of the present study was to investigate IgA anti-jejunal antibody (JAB) in CD children and to compare it with IgG and also with IgA gliadin (AGA) and endomysium (EMA) antibodies. Another aim of the study was to investigate the possible presence of an autoantibody in the disease. A blind study on 175 sera taken from 138 children with malabsorptive syndromes gave the following results: 91% of children with confirmed CD according to ESPGAN criteria had JAB while on a gluten-containing diet, 93% (13/14) of such children before being placed on a gluten-free diet (GFD) and 90% (27/30) on gluten challenge. None of the 21 patients on a GFD for more than one year had JAB. 79% of children with suspected CD with a flat mucosa had JAB: 71% (25/35) of such children who were younger than 2 years, and 94% (16/17) who were older than 2 years.
Neither 53 patients without villous atrophy nor 3 patients with selective IgA deficiency with CD (two) or suspected CD (one) had JAB during gluten intake.
Simultaneous determination of AGA and EMA together with gliadin and tissue absorption studies revealed that AGA is different, EMA is probably identical with JAB.
We suggest that the IgA JAB is the autoantibody of gluten-sensitive enteropathy, detectable as circulating and possible as tissue-deposited antibody.

1. J Invest Dermatol 1986;87:703.
2. Lancet 1971;1:1202.
3. J Invest Dermatol 1988;91:336.
Supported by the Humboldt-Foundation, Bonn, FRG.

EVIDENCE FOR A DOMINANT GENE MECHANISM IN COELIAC DISEASE.

J. Michalski, J. Hernandez, C. McCombs, C. McCarthy, F. Stevens, R. Elston,
LSU Medical Center, New Orleans LA, USA,
University College Hospital, Galway, Ireland.

Although coeliac disease (CD) is strongly associated with the codominantly expressed HLA alleles B8 and DR3, the genetic basis of this illness remains unclear. Recent studies show that at least two unlinked gene loci are involved. A report by Pena et al in 1978 suggested that one of these genes is dominant and the other recessive, but the analysis of Greenberg and Rotter in 1981 did not support a dominant component and instead was consistent with a double recessive gene model.

To address this controversy, we examined the inheritance of CD in 39 families (243 individuals, 61 with CD) from the West of Ireland. HLA-A and B locus alleles were ascertained in all but one of these subjects.

Analysis of the data revealed the following:

1) A significant excess proportion of concordant sib pairs shared two HLA haplotypes whereas an excess proportion of discordant sib pairs had no haplotype in common.
2) Chi square tests confirmed a highly significant association between HLA-B8 and CD (odds-ration=9.394) and a negative association with HLA-B7.
3) Both heterozygotes and homozygotes for HLA-B8 had a significantly increased risk of CD. Homozygotes had a non-significantly greater risk of CD than heterozygotes. We estimate a penetrance of 0.89 for homozygotes and 0.66 for heterozygotes.
4) Using these penetrance estimates, and a prevalence of 1/340 in this population, these data support a one dominant, one recessive, two gene model for the inheritance of CD.

CRYPT INTRAEPITHELIAL LYMPHOCYTES NUMBER IS A SENSITIVE INDEX OF DIETARY COMPLIANCE IN TEENAGER COELIACS.

M. Mayer, R. Troncone, M. Marsh, S. Auricchio. Department of Pediatrics, University of Napels, Italy. University Department of Medicine, Hope Hospital, Salford, Manchester, UK.

Compliance with the gluten-free diet (GFD) is a major problem in certain groups of coeliac patients. Up to 60% of teenagers coeliacs are reported to be off diet. Aims of this study were: 1.to assess compliance with the GFD in a cohort of teenager coeliacs. 2.to assess clinical, immunological and histological consequences of different amounts of gluten present in their diet.

123 Patients were investigated (mean age 13.7 yrs; range 11-23). The amount of dietary gluten, symptoms, associated diseases were assessed; antigliadin antibodies (AGA) were measured. 36 Patients underwent a jejunal biopsy; a morphometric evaluation was carried out by a computerised image analysis sytem.

80 Patients (65%) resulted to be on a GFD (group A); 29 (23.5%) on a normal diet (average daily gluten content: 15g) (group B); 14 (11.5%) on a semistrict diet (average daily gluten content: 0.73g; range 0.06-2) (group C). Standardised height was not different in the three groups, weight was heavier in group A. Gastrointestinal symptoms were significantly more represented in group B but not in group C, when compared to group A. Raised AGA levels were noted in 17%, 25% and 14% of patients in group A, B and C, respectively. A decrease of surface epithelial volume and surface intraepithelial lymphocytes (IEL), an increase of crypt epithelial volume and crypt IEL were observed in group B patients when compared to group A. In group C, patients showed an increase of crypt volume and crypt IEL; once excluded 4 cases with gross histological alterations, the absolute number of crypt IEL persisted significantly increased.

In conclusion, 65% of our teenager coeliacs was compliant with a strict GFD. Clinical symptoms and AGA levels did not help in assessing compliance. Patients ingesting small amounts of gluten (less than 1 g daily) showed increased absolute number of crypt IEL. These data suggest that small amounts of gluten are able to activate mucosal cell-mediated immunity, and may represent a potential risk for coeliac patients. A strict gluten-free diet is mandatory.

UPPER G.I. DAMAGES SEEN AT ENDOSCOPY IN CHILDREN WITH COELIAC DISEASE.

G. Oderda, M. Forni, P. Lerro, E. Poli, K. Tavassoli, N. Ansaldi. Paediatric Gastroenterology, University of Turin, Italy.

Endoscopic duodenal biopsies to diagnose Coeliac Disease (CD) can be easily obtained with forceps. AIM: to study mucosal damages seen during gastroscopy performed to obtain duodenal biopsies, and their relation to a gluten containing diet in childhood CD.

Since 1985 we performed 157 gastroscopies in 108 children (age range 1 to 23 yrs, 37 males) with CD. In the active phase on a gluten containing diet in 12 pts, after 6 months of Gluten Free Diet (GFD) in 34, after gluten challenge in 55, after a second gluten challenge in 39, and to monitor a GFD in 17. Gastroscopies were always performed with a paediatric endoscope (Olympus XP20) after a mild sedation with oral diazepam, and biopsies were obtained with paediatric forceps with open cup diameter of 5 mm. Upper G.I. damages were seen in 113 cases (72%) and confirmed by histological examination in 43 (27%); they were significantly more frequent in children on a gluten containing diet than on a GFD ($p<.001$.). Most frequent endoscopic damages were: duodenitis (52 of 155 = 33%) and oesophagitis (50 of 155 = 32%). Most frequent changes at histology were: duodenal atrophy in 121 pts on gluten diet and oesophagitis in 17 pts (11%). Oesophagitis was significantly more frequent in children on a gluten diet ($p<.05$), and its frequence increased significantly with duration of gluten challenge and with advancing age, but a causal relationship between gluten and oesophagitis could not be established. In patients with mucosal damages, symptomes (abdominal pain or recurrent vomiting) were more frequent ($p<.01$). In all patients we obtained at least one duodenal biopsy satisfactory for histological examination.

CONCLUSION: In children with CD upper G.I. mucosa can be damaged in areas other than the duodenum. Gastroscopy, performed to obtain duodenal biopsy, can give additional information useful for CD patient management.

HLA CLASS II CONTRIBUTION TO COELIAC DISEASE -A FAMILY STUDY-

W.J. Bolsover, M.A. Hall, P.J. Ciclitira,
Dep. of Paediatrics and Pharmacology,
UMDS Guys & St. Thomas's Hospitals, London, UK.

There is an association between coeliac disease (CD) and markers throughout the MHC class II region, particularly with HLA-DR3, DR7, DQw2 and DPw1. We wished to investigate this further by determining the coinheritance of these alleles with CD amongst members of multiply affected families. 13 Families with 2 or more patients were identified. Peripheral blood DNA was extracted from affected individuals and all available first degree relatives. The DNA was digested with Taq I, Bgl II, Msp I, Rsa I and Xba I endonucleases and subjected to Southern blot analysis with HLA-DRB, DQA, DQB, DPA and DPB cDNA probes.

112 Individuals including 34 coeliacs were studied. All the affected individuals were HLA- DR3, DQw2. Eleven of them were HLA-DR3, DR7 and 12 were HLA- DR3 homozygous; both these combinations were significantly more frequent than in a control group ($p<0.05$). Twenty-six of the 34 (76%) were HLA-DPw1 compared with 24% of HLA-DR3 controls ($p<0.01$) while 33 had the previously described Rsa I/DPB 4.0 kb band. All the affected members within 12 of the families shared an HLA-B8, DR3, DQw2 haplotype, 8 of which included HLA-DPw1. Only 10 of these 12 families were informative for the 4.0 kb Rsa I/DPB band, which was co-inherited with HLA-DR3 in 8 out of 10. In 1 family the 2 affected members shared HLA-DRw7, DQw2 and DPw1, each with a different HLA-B8, DR3, DQw2 haplotype. The association between CD and various HLA-DP markers appeared to be secondary to the linkage between the latter and DR3. CD was present in 32 of the 63 individuals who had the disease-associated HLA-B8, DR3, DQw2 haplotype.

The results confirm an association of CD with HLA-B8, DR3, DQw2 and DPw1, the latter representing part of an extended MHC haplotype. They suggest that a specific HLA gene product is necessary, but insufficient alone, for the development of CD. Further investigation of these individual alleles by DNA sequencing should clarify which MHC class II genes are responsible. This would enable easier identification of indiviuals at risk.

DIABETES-RELATED IMMUNOLOGIC MARKERS IN CHILDREN COELIAC DISEASE.

M. Bonamico, G. Ballati, P. Mariani, M. Morellini, R. Perfetti, E. Anastasi, U. Di Mario. Dep. of Pediatrics, Experimental Medicine, Endocrinology University, "La Sapienza" - Rome - Italy.

The pathogenesis of coeliac disease (CD) is still obscure despite a growing body of evidence suggesting a role for immunological abnormalities in the sequence of causative events. A clinical association between CD and type I diabetes (DM1) has been reported. Therefore, in addition to antigliadin antibodies (AGA), CD children HLA typed were also tested for humoral immune factors, known to be related to DM1: serum anti-insulin (IAAb) and - immunoglobulin (αIgAb) autoantibodies, anti-islet cell antibodies (ICA) and anti-glucagon antibodies.
Fifteen children with CD on gluten containing diet (Group 1) have been recruited together with: 15 coeliac patients following a gluten-free-diet (Group 2), 16 children with irritable gut (Group 3) and 14 children with no gastrointestinal symptoms (Group 4) as controls. There was a significant association between CD and HLA-DR3 ($p<0.001$) and/or DR7 ($p<0.05$) when compared to a cross-matched population. AGA-IgA were present in all patients of Group 1, in two patients of Group 2 and in one patient of Group 3 children; similarly, AGA IgG were present in all patients of Group 1, in two patients of Group 2 and in two patients of Group 3. IAAb were present in 27% of Group 1 and in 20% Group 2 patients. αIgAb were significantly increased in Group 1 and 2 in comparison with both Group 3 and 4; two patients in Group 2 were positive for ICA and none for anti-glucagon antibodies. The levels of αIgAb in Group 1 were positively correlated with AGA ($r=0.49$). No clear association was found between HLA antigens and antibody presence.
In this study diabetes related immune factors have been shown to be present in a number of coeliac children in absence of clinical symptoms of diabetes. Surprisingly, this positivity of diabetes-related autoantibodies remained substantially unchanged in children on a gluten-free-diet while AGA tend to normalize. Thus, CD and DM1 in addition to a partly common genetic background, seem to share other immunopathogenetic mechanisms.

HLA ANTIGENS AND PHENOTYPES ASSOCIATED WITH SEVERE IMMUNOGLOBULIN - A DEFICIENCY IN COELIAC DISEASE PAEDIATRIC PATIENTS.

N. Clerici, M. Fernandez, I. Polanco. Dep. of Immunologia, Hospital Ramón y Cajal, Unyt of Gastroenterology. Children Hospital "La Paz" - Madrid - Spain.

Class I and II HLA antigens were determined by a standard microlymphocytotoxicity test in 45 paediatric patients with severe Immunoglobulin A deficiency (serum levels of IgA <5mg/dl) and in all first degree relatives of eighteen of them. IgG and IgM serum levels were normal in almost all patients and in all members of the families. This study included two subgroups of IgA deficient (IgA-d) patients: one (CD) composed by 12 coeliac patients (8 girls and 4 boys, mean age at the time of diagnosis (DMA: 3.3) and the other (RTIAG) of 33 patients (22 boys and 11 girls, DMA: 5.7) with frequent respiratory tract infections, allergic diseases or gastrointestinal disorders. It was found that the HLA antigens associated with IgA deficiency were different from one subgroup to the other. When HLA antigen frequencies in IgA-d coeliac patients were compared with those present in 51 CD children with normal serum levels of IgA, the frequency of B14 was found to be significantly increased among IgA-d (36.4% vs 7.8%, $p=4.0x10^{-2}$) and resulted in an elevated relative risk: RR=6.71 and etiological fraction: EF=0.31. Among RTIAG patients: the frequency of DR1 antigen was significantly raised when compared with those of 166 healthy local donors (63.3%, $p=2.1x10^{-4}$, RR=5.47, EF=0.52). Frequencies of phenotypes: DR1,DR3; B35,DR1; A28,B14,DR1 were also increased with RR of 7.01; 4.96 and 11.10 respectively. Despite the differences found, similarities were observed between both groups of patients: the increasing frequencies of shared phenotypes A1,B8,DR3 and DR1, DR3 and the negative association of DR2 and DR4 antigens. These findings strongly suggest that HLA region gene(s) may be involved in the susceptibility of IgA deficiency and allele of different loci could be related according to the type of associated disease. We conclude that the presence of B14 could increase the risk in coeliac disease and DR1 could play a similar role in patients with respiratory, allergic or gastrointestinal pathologies.

DR3 AND DR7 -NEGATIVE COELIAC DISEASE (CD)- A CLINICALLY RELEVANT ENTITY?

B. Winklhofer-Roob, E. Rossipal, D.H. Shmerling, G. Granditsh, G. Lanzer, A. Hajek- Rosenmayr, E. Albert, M. Decurtins.
Dept.of Paediatrics, Univ. Graz, Zurich, Vienna, Munich Tissue Typing Laboratories, Dept. Internal Medicine, Univ. Graz Inst. of Blood Group Serology, Univ. Vienna Dept. of Surgery, Univ. Zürich

The association of CD with B8, DR3, DR7 and DQw2 is well known. However, little is known whether the lack of these antigens in CD patients (2-32%) is clinically relevant. To determine whether there is any heterogeneity in the clinical presentation and course up to this investigation, a retrospective study was conducted.
Of 403 HLA-typed CD patients from 3 pediatric clinics, 20 were negative for both DR3 and DR7, as well as for B8 and with one exception for DQw2. In these patients, DR4 (45%) and DR5 (70%) were significantly more frequent compared with the remaining patients (DR4:7%, DR5:27%) and with controls negative for both DR3 and DR7 (DR4:18%, DR5:30%).
The diagnosis of CD was established by the evidence of a flat mucosa and a clinical improvement on an gluten free diet. Age at weaning (median; range (months) 0.75; 0.00-4.50), age at introduction of gluten (4.50; 2.00-6.50), duration of the free intervall (1.50; 0.00-13.50), age at first symptoms (6.87; 3.00-17.00) and age at diagnosis (8.50; 5.0-23.75) did not differ significantly from the other CD patients.
In the initial clinical presentation, some features were more frequent in the DR3-DR7-negative subgroup (diarrhea: 75% vs 53%, abdominal pain: 11% vs 1%, muscular hypotonia: 8% vs 1%) and others were less (constipation: 0% vs 4%) as compared with the remaining ones. However, with regard to the known variability of symptoms in CD the differences are not significant. Laboratory findings (anemia, iron deficiency, hypoproteinemia, hypoprothrombinemia, hypocholesterolemia) also showed no significant difference.
The further course of these patients (permanence of gluten intolerance, malignancy) will show whether this subgroup of patients represents a clinical entity or otherwise is to be considered as irrelevant.

INTESTINAL EXPRESSION OF HLA-DQ ALLELES ASSOCIATED TO COELIAC DISEASE

J.J. Schweizer, M.L. Mearin, A.S. Peña, G.J.A. Offerhaus, B.O. Roep, R.E. Bontrop, L.J. Dooren, C.B.H.W. Lamers, Ph.J. Hoedemaecker. Depts. Paediatrics, Gastroenterology, Pathology, Immunology, University Hospital Leiden, TNO Primate Center, Rijswijk, The Netherlands.

Studies at DNA and product level of B cell lines of coeliac patients have shown a strong association between coeliac disease (CD) and the HLA-DQα2.3 and HLA-DQβ2.7 alleles. The antisera monoclonals SFR20-DQα5 and XIII-358.4, which specifically react with the HLA-DQα2.3 and with the HLA-DQβ2.3 and -DQβ2.7 respectively, have been used to detect the expression of these specificities in the small intestine mucosa of 7 coeliac patients and 11 non-coeliac persons. An immunoperoxidase technique on frozen tissue sections of jejunal biopsy specimens was used. Positive specimens showed immunoperoxidase staining of lymphocytes and histiocytes in the lamina propria. The epithelial cells showed no immunoperoxidase staining. Positive results at the intestinal level correlated with the HLA-typing of the patients and controls. The distribution found for the HLA-DQ alleles in the intestinal mucosa of coeliac patients makes the role of a HLA-DQα/β dimer as gliadin receptor at the epithelial cell less probable, but supports the hypothesis that these DQ molecules are involved in the regulation of the intestinal immune response to gluten.

IS PERSISTENT ADENOVIRUS 12 (Ad12) INFECTION INVOLVED IN COELIAC DISEASE?

P. Howdle, J. Mahon, B. Scott, G. Wood, M. Losowsky, G. Blair, Depts. Med., St. James's University Hospital, Dep. Biochem., Leeds University, Leeds, U.K.

An amino acid sequence homology between gliadin and the E1B-58kDa protein of Ad12 led to the hypothesis that prior infection with Ad12 could lead to the development of CD, probably as a result of immunological cross-reactivity. Coeliac patients have an increased titre of Ad12 neutralising antibody but not of specific anti-E1B-58kDa antibody. They also have evidence of cell-mediated immunity to synthetic peptides corresponding to the amino acid sequences implicated. We sought evidence of persistent Ad12 infection by analysing DNA from small intestinal mucosa using the Polymerase chain reaction with specific oligonucleotide probes designed to amplify the region of the Ad12 E1B gene involved. Duodenal biopsies were obtained from 24 controls (mean age 41, range 9-70, 12 males) and 18 coeliac patients (7 untreated, mean age 49, range 23-73, 10 males). Specific PCR amplified products were detected in 3 coeliac patients, 1 untreated and 2 controls (N.S. Fisher's Exact Test). We conclude that coeliac patients do not have an increased incidence of persistent Ad12 infection. Cross-reactivity between gliadin and the E1B-58kDa protein could still be a pathogenetic factor in CD but our findings bring into question the proposed hypothesis since we have shown no direct link between CD and persistent Ad12 infection.

NEGATIVE HUMORAL RESPONSE TO ADENOVIRUS 12 IN COELIAC DISEASE.

L.A. Dieleman, A.S. Peña, H. van Doorninck, M.L. Mearin, W. van Duijn, C.B.H.W. Lamers, Depts. of Gastroenterology and Paediatrics, Leiden University Hosptial, Leiden, The Netherlands.

It has been suggested that an encounter of the immune system with antigenic determinants produced during intestinal Ad12 viral infection may be important in the pathogenesis of coeliac disease (CD).
The aim of our study was to investigate the frequency of antibodies directed against this region in the sera of patients with CD, in order to assess the possible significance of this finding in the pathogenesis of the disease. Serum antibodies to sonicated Ad12- and Ad5-transformed baby rabbit kidney cells were assayed by an IgG immunoblotting technique (IgG-IB). No reaction against this 54 kD band after blotting with sera obtained from 23 patients with CD with high and low antigliadin antibodies was found. These findings suggest that the humoral crossreactivity between the homologous E1B-54 kD protein of Ad12 and the A-gliadin molecule does not play an important role in the pathogenesis of CD in the group of patients sofar studied. These findings do not rule out the role of humoral crossreactivity in other populations. The technique reported here which is cheaper than radioimmuno-assay analysis can be easily applied to the study of larger group of patiens.

CHARACTERIZATION OF γδ TCR IN T CELL CLONES FROM SMALL INTESTINE OF COELIAC DISEASE PATIENTS.

G. De Libero, G. Casorati, M.P. Rocci, G. Oderda, K. Tavassoli, A. Lanzavecchia, N. Migone. Basel Institute for Immunology, Dipartimento di Genetica, Biologia e Chimica Medica, Cattedra di Pediatria, University of Torino.

We have isolated T cell lines and clones from jejunal intestinal biopsies and peripheral blood of 7 coeliac disease (CD) patients, and 5 controls. T cells, expanded in the presence of PHA, rhIL-2 and feeder cells, were stained with the following mAbs: TR66 (anti-CD3), BMA032 (anti-αβ TCR), δ1 (anti-δ chain), δTCS1 (anti-Vδ1/Jδ1), BB3 (anti-Vδ2), TiγA (anti-Vγ9), C4-4A11 (anti-Vγ4), anti-CD4, and anti-CD8. The analysis of T cell lines showed that γδ+ cells are increased in the gut of CD patients (range 15-52%) when compared to the controls (3-15%). Vδ1 was the most represented Vδ chain (47-76% of total γδ cells), while Vδ2 was always below 21%. Vδ1 and Vδ2 negative γδ cells were 11-42%. Vγ9 ranged from 18-68%, while Vγ4 varied between 14 and 41%. On the contrary, gut-γδ cells derived from controls showed a higher variability in the Vδ and Vγ gene usage.
In the peripheral blood of the patients, γδ cells were only a minor population (<10%) neverthless the Vδ1, Vδ2 and Vγ9, Vγ4 gene usage appeared to correlate to what found in the gut. Analysis of 91 gut clones from 4 donors did not show a preferential pairing of Vδ1 with Vγ9 nor with Vγ4. Molecular analysis of Vδ1 and Vδ2 negative cell subset showed a predominant expression of Vδ3 (7 out of 9 CD analyzed clones were Vδ3+). These results, together with our previous studies in thymus and peripheral blood (J.Exp.Med.1989;170:1521), suggest that Vδ3 is more represented in the gut than in thymus and peripheral blood and that is more frequent in γδ cells from CD patients than in normal gut.
The higher frequency of γδ cells and their particular V gene usage in CD as compared to controls suggests that these cells might play a role in the disease. We are currently attempting to identify the specificities of γδ cells in CD patients.

CHARACTERIZATION OF INTESTINAL $\tau\delta$ AND $\alpha\beta$ T-CELL RECEPTOR POSITIVE CELLS IN COELIAC DISEASE.

C.J.J. Rust, A.S. Peña, Ph.M. Kluin, F. Koning, Depts. of Immunohaematology & Bloodbank, Gastoenterology and Pathology, Academic Hospital, Leiden, The Netherlands.

Histo-immunological analysis of jejunum biopsies from patients with coeliac disease (CD) has demonstrated that $\alpha\beta$ T-cells are mainly present in the lamina propria whereas $\tau\delta$ T-cells can be detected predominantly in the epithelium. To investigate the function of intestinal T-cells, we isolated T-cells from jejunum biopsies and expanded thes in vitro. In such cultures significant percentages of $\tau\delta$ T-cells were present (up to 26%) whereas in other cultures, of patients with unrelated gut diseases, no or very little $\tau\delta$ t-cells were detected. From two patients with CD $\tau\delta$ and $\alpha\beta$ T-cell clones haave been generated from the bulk cultures. These T-cell clones have been characterized by FACS analysis and SDS-PAGE analysis of the TCR's. Variability was observed with regard to the expression of CD5, CD7 and CD8 markers on $\tau\delta$ T-cells (no CD4 $\tau\delta$ T-cells could be detected) and the use of τ and δ V-regions, indicating that intestinal $\tau\delta$ T-cells are a heterogeneous set of cells. Functional analysis of the T-cell clones will be carried out using a testsystem in which autologous EBV transformed B-cells will be used as antigen presenting cells. These cells will be cultured for several days with α-gliadin. Both the $\alpha\beta$ and $\tau\delta$ T-cell clones will be tested for proliferation to and killing of the α-gliadin pulsed B-cells. These experiments are in preparation.

INTERCELLULAR ADHESION MOLECULE-1 EXPRESSION IN COELIAC DISEASE

R.P. Sturgess, J.C. Macartney, J.M. Nelufer, M.W. Makgoba, P.J. Ciclitira, Divisions of Pharmacology and Medicine, The Rayne Institu, UMDS, St. Thomas'London & Division of Molecular Endocrinology, RPMS, Hammersmith Hospital, London UK.

Coeliac disease (CD) is characterised by a gluten induced damage to the small intestinal mucosa in genetically predisposed individuals that is thought to be immune mediated. Intercellular adhesion molecule-1 (ICAM-1) mediates a variety of cell-cell interactions in immunity and inflammation by binding to the leucocyte adhesion receptor molecule LFA-1. We investigated the expression of ICAM-1 on jejunal biopsies from patients with untreated and treated CD and have explored the role of antigen in modulating this expression, by gluten challenge. Peroral jejunal biopsies were taken from controls (n=7), treated (n=10) and untreated (n=9) CD patients. Three patients with treated disease underwent jejunal biopsy prior to and half hourly for six hours after gluten challenge.
Frozen sections were examined immunohistochemically using a streptavidin-biotin immunoperoxidase method with the monoclonal antibody 84H10 against ICAM-1. There was no staining of the intra-epithelial lymphocytes or the epithelial enterocytes in biopsies from any of the patients. There was universal staining of endothelial cells in biopsies from all the patients. The biopsies from the untreated CD patients exhibited significantly greater staining of the superficial lamina propria cells than in controls ($p<0.01$) and those from the treated CD group ($p<0.05$). Gluten challenge induced increased ICAM-1 expression within two hours in the treated patients in a similar pattern of distribution to that found in the untreated patients. We believe this to be the first human, in vivo, demonstration of the kinetics, and differential upregulation of ICAM-1 expression at the site of an inflammatory response and is evidence of an immunomodulatory role for ICAM-1 in the pathogenesis of CD. Increased expression of ICAM-1 on the superficial lamina propria population of cells from untreated CD patients compared to controls provides further evidence for the role of activated T-lymphocytes in the pathogenesis of CD.

COELIAC DISEASE IN CYPRUS

J.M. Hadjiminas, N. Persianis, M. Angastiniotis, J.A. Walker-Smith. Cyprus Paediatric Society, Nicosia, Cyprus, Dep. Paediatrics, Makarios III Hospital, Nicosia, Cyprus, Dep. of Paediatric Gastroenterology, St Bartholomews Hospital, London, UK.

There is currently no published report of coeliac disease (CD) in the Greek Cypriot population. Four cases are described.

Case 1. An 18 month old boy was seen with diarrhoea, abdominal distension and failure to thrive. Small bowel biopsy was consistent with CD. Anti-gliadin antibodies were positive. There was a dramatic response to gluten free diet and the child is now 3 years old and well.

Case 2. A 22 month old boy with diarrhoea, abdominal distension and failure to thrive had a small bowel biopsy consistent with CD. He responded well to gluten free diet and is now 1 month after starting his diet, gaining weight and free of diarrhoea.

Case 3. An 18 month old boy with failure to thrive and diarrhoea had a small bowel biopsy consistent with CD. He is now well at the age of 9 years and continues his diet.

Case 4. A two year old boy with chronic diarrhoea had a small bowel biopsy consistent with CD. He responded well to gluten free diet.

The prevailing impression that CD is rare in Cyprus is in our opinion mistaken. The current practice of placing children on gluten free diet often in combination with milk free diet without prior investigation including small bowel biopsy is to be condemned. We feel that proper investigation would lead to the diagnosis and correct management of a number of cases now missed.

COELIAC DISEASE IN SAUDI CHILDREN

Hisham Nazer, Nadia Sakati & Harb Harfi. Dep. of Pediatrics, King Faisal Specialist Hospital and Research Centre, Riyadh 11311, Saudi Arabia

Coeliac Disease (CD) is a recognised cause of chronic diarrhoea and growth retardation in infancy and childhood. Therefore, it presents an important challenge to clinicians, especially those working in the developing countries where chronic diarrhoea poses a major health hazard.
This report is to confirm the existence of coeliac disease in Saudi Arabia and to highlight the delay in its diagnosis. Twenty two Saudi children were diagnosed to have CD over the period of 1978-1988. They were referred with growth retardation and abdominal distention. History of chronic diarrhoea was present in 21 children and recurrent vomiting in 13. Mean age at onset of symptoms was 1.9 years (range 0.3-11), at referral 3.4 years (0.4-11.5), at diagnosis 5.9 years (0.9-16), with a mean delay in diagnosis of 2.8 years (0.2-11).
Intestinal biopsies were obtained in 21 cases. The remaining case had its initial biopsy abroad. Sixteen patients had evidence of severe mucosal injury (flat mucosa) and six patients had partial villous atrophy. Fifteen children responded well to gluten-free diet (GFD). Intestinal biopsies were obtained from ten children with evidence of histological remission in seven. Poor compliance to GFD contributed to the lack of favourable response in three children with evidence of histological relapse in two. Clinical relapse within two years following gluten challenge was reported in all eight cases studied; five of them also had histological relapse. It is concluded that the relatively low prevalence of CD in Saudi Arabia may be due to failure of diagnosis. Poor compliance to GFD explains the high rate of nonresponse among children with CD. A higher index of suspicion for the diagnosis of CD in Saudi Arabia is needed.

THE SPECTRUM OF GLUTEN INTOLERANCE IN A DEFINED PAEDIATRIC POPULATION

J.F.B. Dossetor, J. Little, D. Eakins. Dep. of Paediatrics, Queen Elizabeth Hospital, Norfolk, UK.

Over a period of nine years from a population of 32.950 children under fifteen, thirty-two children responded to a gluten free diet. Almost all children underwent jejunal biopsy before being put on the gluten free diet. Two children moved into the area on gluten free diets already with the diagnosis made elsewhere. Reviewing the clinical and biopsy changes of the remaining thrirty, the children fall into three groups. The first group (6) comprises children who fit the description of classical coeliac disease with subtotal or partial villous atrophy and a characteristic history. The second group (18) comprises children with what is usually known as wheat intolerance with minimal biopsy change, rapid reactions to wheat, and often other food atopic reactions. A third group (6) consists of children with minimal biopsy change and deceptive histories. It is possible that this group would become more classical coeliacs with further exposure to gluten. The different biopsy features of the three groups are reviewed.
The Health District in question is comparatively isolated and most symptomatic children would have been seen at the one hospital. Knowing the size of the childhood population served it is possible to calculate approximate incidences for the three varieties of gluten intolerance for this population of children.

THE REASONS OF MALNUTRITION IN CHILDREN WITH COELIAC DISEASE

J. Socha, J. Rujner, H. Gregorek, A. Stolarczyk, G. Lyson, B. Muszunska, E. Kulesza, A. Kowalik, K. Madalinski. Child Health Center, Warsaw, Poland.

The aim of study was to estimate the reasons of malnutrition in children with coeliac disease:
1. Errors of nourishment
2. Excessive content of gluten in "gluten free diet"
3. Social causes.

Methods: The study was carried out in 190 patients (pts) from 3 to 16 years, 107 who complied with gluten free diet (eg with normal mucosa) and 83 pts. who didn't comply with diet (flat mucosa).

The following parameters were estimated:
1. Nutritional status: anthropometrical, densitometry of bons, biochemical tests (Hb, Alb, Fe, vit.A, E, 25OHD3).
2. The way of nourishment (history of nourishment during last 2 weeks and anamnesis of nourishment in the last 24 hours).
3. Gluten concentration in "gluten free diet" (ELISA*).
4. The social causes:
   a. check up of mothers knownledge about pathogenesis and therapy of coeliac disease (12 standard questions).
   b. inquiries concerning material and social problems of the family, medical care and other insitutions.

Result: The pts. who did not comply with the diet were often malnourished (lower body fat mass), in 25% concentration of 25OHD3 below 10 ug/ml and in 45% vit.A below 300 ug/ml. Inproper nourishment were stated mainly among older children. It concerned frequency of feeding, quality composition of diet especially deficiency of carbohydrate and higher consumption of protein and animal fat. There are some main factors which are cause of failure in treatment:
1. Too high concentration of gluten in gluten free diet (above 10 ug/g of product).
2. The high correlation between mothers knowledge about the disease and compliance with diet was found. Compliance with diet did not depend on age of parents and pts., material status of family, other chronic illness in family etc.

Conclusion:
1. Main factor which decides about compliance with diet is the mothers knowledge of disease especially about therapy.
2. The gluten content in "gluten free diet" can be too high for some patients.

* Authors are greateful Prof. Hekkens for introducing his method in our Insitute.

NERVOUS SYSTEM INVOLVEMENT IN PAEDIATRIC COELIAC PATIENTS

B. Papadatou, M. Di Capua, M. Gambarara, G. Castellucci, V. Lucidi, F. Ferretti, A.M. Colombo, S. Bella, M. Castro. Divisione di Gastroenterologia, Ospedale Bambino Gesù Roma Divisione di Neurologia Ospedale Bambino Gesù Roma Clinica Pediatrica Università Perugia.

In some patients, coeliac disease (CD) is associated with clinical dysfunction of the nervous system, expressed variably as encephalopathy, cerebellar syndrome, seizures, epilepsy with occipital calcifications, psychiatric disorders, myelopathy, myopathy and periferal neuropathy. Such dysfunctions are described in adult patients generally within 10 years after the diagnosis. Recently the association of CD and epilepsy with occipital calcifications has been reported in few pediatric patients. The pathogenesis of nervous system involvement is unkown; disorders in immune mechanisms caused by CD and vitamin deficiencies (vit.E, B12, B6, folic acid) are involved. The following report describes two girls with CD who during gluten-free diet developed one a type of distal axonic degeneration and the other a leukoencephalopathy.

The first case refers to a 6 years old girl with CD that was diagnosed at 11 months of age and then confirmed at 4 years of age following ESPGAN protocol. During gluten- free diet she developed weakness of the legs, positive Gowers, Areflexia; the gait was wide-based and there was impaired perception of touch, pain and temperature in stocking distribution. The EMG showed a picture like that of a distal axonic neuropathy. Somatosensory evoked potentials were normal. Her cerebrospinal fluid was normal and the research of neuropathy viruses was negative. Vitamin E and B12 plasma levels resulted normal. In spite of normal vitamin levels the girl was treated with parenteral administration of vitamin E for 4 months. In the next 18 months a slow improvement was observed. A new EMG was normal.

The second case refers to a 14 years old girl with CD that was diagnosed at 13 years of age, who during gluten-free diet presented fever, weakness and spinal pain. Speech was scanning. The ocular fundi and cranial nerve functions were normal. Strenght was normal, lasegue positive and there was a contraction of paravertebral muscles. Spinal fluid exam showed a light increase of proteins and white cells. Cranial CT scan showed aereas of hypodensity in parietal-temporal lobes of both hemispheres and cerebral MRI showed demyelination in the same aereas.

Antigliadin antibodies were absent, the research of neurotropy viruses was negative and plasma levels of vitamins E and B12 were normal. The girl was treated with prednisone 2 mgr/Kgr for 1 month with slow improvement. Symptoms disappeared after six months. Three years later the clinical remission continues. Our cases show that an axonic neuropathy and a leukoencephalopathy can also affect pediatric patients with CD on gluten-free diet within a short time after diagnosis.

COELIAC DISEASE AND EPILEPSY WITH POSTERIOR CEREBRAL CALCIFICATIONS: A CAUSAL ASSOCIATION.

M. Gilda Zaniboni, A. Lambertini, N. Romeo, A. Licignano, P. Ambrosetto, G. Gobbi. Dept.of Pediatrics, Ospedale Maggiore, Bologna - Italy. Dept.of Child Neurology, Medical School, University of Bologna - Italy.

Eight patients (4 males, 4 females) affected by epilepsy with cerebral calcifications mainly located in the posterior region were subjected to a battery of tests including an intestinal biopsy. Our aim was to find out whether or not all of the patients also suffered from coeliac disease (CD). CD was found in 6 of the 8 patients tested. This result together with other individual cases reported in the literature suggests that the triad of diseases (epilepsy, posterior cerebral calcifications and CD) are causally related. Folate deficiencies, present only in the cases of malabsorption and absent in the others, did not appear to be a determining factor for the presence of calcifications. The possibility that the calcifications were due to the Sturge-Weber syndrome was also excluded and hence their etiology remains unknown. The same HLA phenotype was found in all the 8 patients, including the 2 cases without coeliac disease. This suggests that a disorder of the immune system lies at the basis of these diseases. Our results suggest that particular attention should be paid to the search for CD in all patients with epilepsy and cerebral calcifications. Further genetic studies are needed to better understand the role played by genetic factors in the etiopathogenesis of these multifactorial diseases.

GENETIC AND IMMUNOLOGICAL MARKERS IN CHILDREN WITH DERMATITIS HERPETIFORMIS

C. Barbera, A. Amoroso, S. Bundino, M. Vallati, P. Fusco, C. Mazzola, N. Ansaldi.
Dep. of Paediatrics, Genetics, Dermathology University of Turin-Italy.

The close link between Dermatitis Herpetiformis (DH) and Coeliac Disease (CD) is well known. Rash in DH is gluten dependent and an enteropathy is found in one majorithy of patients. Both diseases share similar genetic markers. In our population the following HLA antigens were significantly associated with DH (in brackets the relative risk): A1 (2.2) B8 (6.2) Cw7 (3.9) DR3 (5.2) DR7 (4.4) Rw53 (4.7) DQw2 (6.0). A diagnosis of jejunal damage (without biopsy) is more difficult in DH in respect to CD because in general clinical symptoms do not correlate to the degree and extent of lesions which may be patchy. It is therefore essential to identify a specific test for the diagnosis and follow up of the disease. Aim of the work was to compare the occurrence of three immunological markers, two extensively used for the diagnosis of CD and DH (antigliadin AGA and antireticulin ARA) to a more recently proposed one antiendomysial antibody EmA, in order to evaluate the sensibility and specificity of the different tests. The results in the table demonstrate in percentages the antibody reactions in DH, CD and in the control group; titers of antibodies correlate well with the mucosal status in DH.

	IgG AGA	IgA ARA	IgA EmA
Patients	Elisa	IFL	IFL
Normal diet	37% 13/35	69.6% 23/33	90.9% 30/33
DH gfd?	0%	0%	0%
Normal diet	85.4% 41/48	88.4% 122/138	92.6% 25/27
CD gfd?	20% 28/140	5.6% 4/71	30% 3/10
Controls	0%	0.5%	0%

THE CLINICAL USE OF THE GLIADIN ANTIBODY TEST

B.W.E. van der Meer, M.L. Mearin, A.S. Peña, C.B.H.W. Lamers, J.L. Dooren. Depts. of Paediatrics and Gastroenterology, University Hospital, Leiden, The Netherlands.

Screeningtests for coeliac disease (CD) can be used to find the patients who should go for a small intestine biopsy. The presence of high gliadin antibodies in serum has been rapported as a good screeningsmethod for CD. We have retrospectively studied the clinical use of the antigliadin antibody test with an ELISA technique on 257 children seen between January 1987 and December 1988 at the Childrens Department of the Leiden University Hospital. In 53 cases it was possible to study the correlation between the pathological findings of the small intestine and the results of the gliadin antibody titers in serum. We conclude that the gliadin antibodies test as screeningsmethod for CD must be based on the measurement of the total immunoglobulines - as well as on the IgA- and IgG-antibodies. Normal titers make the diagnosis CD less probable. High gliadin antibody titers in serum are not diagnostic for CD but they form an indication to perform a small intestine biopsy.

SERUM ANTIGLIADIN ANTIBODIES DURING GLUTEN CHALLENGE

E.A.K. Wauters, R.H.J. Houwen, Th. Ockhuizen. Wilhelmina Childrens Hospital, Utrecht, The Netherlands. TNO-CIVO, Zeist, The Netherlands.

Coeliac disease (CD) is defined as a permanent intolerance to gluten, resulting in total atrophy of jejunal villi. A gluten provocation test, with a jejunal biopsy before and after the challenge, is necessary to assess the permanency of this condition. A non-invasive method to asses the mucosal integrity during gluten challenge might enhance the acceptance of this provocation test by patients and their parents. The serial measurement of antigliadin antibodies (AGA) during gluten challenge could be such a method, because the AGA concentration seems to correlate with gluten intake in CD. Therefore we compared the histology of the small intestinal mucosa with the concentration of serum AGA-IgG and AGA-IgA before and at the end of the gluten challenge in 17 patients with suspected CD. Serum AGA-IgG and AGA-IgA were determined using an ELISA technique and concentrations were expressed in arbitrary units (AU). In 111 random blood samples the mean + 3SD for AGA-IgG was 120 AU and for AGA-IgA was 4 AU. In 7 out of 17 children the histological appearance of the intestinal mucosa was unaffected by the gluten challenge, while in 10 children villus atrophy indicated a persisting gluten intolerance. In all children with villus atrophy a marked increase in AGA was observed, exceeding the normal mean + 3SD for both IgG and IgA (122-1144 AU and 10-115 AU respectively). In the children with a normal jejunal histology the AGA concentrations remained within normal ranges (AGA-IgG 9-70 AU, AGA-IgA 1-3 AU). We conclude that serum AGA during gluten challenge are sensitive markers of mucosal damage and could replace jejunal biopsies.

IgG-SUBCLASS ANTIBODIES TO FOOD ANTIGENS IN PATIENTS WITH COELIAC DISEASE

M. Hvatum, H. Scott, P. Brandtzaeg. Lab. Immunohistochemistry and Immunopathology (LIIPAT) Rikshospitalet, Oslo, Norway.

The subclass pattern of serum IgG antibodies to antigens from wheat, oat, soya, cow's milk and egg was studied by an ELISA in 14 adults with coeliac disease (CD) and in 10 controls with other intestinal disorders. Despite the low level of IgG4 in normal serum (only 0.7-5% of total IgG), the IgG activity to β-lactoglobulin was mainly expressed by IgG4 (median 75%). The IgG4 activity to α-lactalbumin and ovalbumin was also relatively high, both in CD (52% and 55%, respectively) and in controls (83% and 82%, respectively). The IgG subclass pattern to gliadin and casein varied considerably in both groups. The IgG4 activity to gliadin was significantly lower ($p<0.02$) in the CD group than in the controls. IgG1 (or IgG1+IgG3) activity to gliadin was often dominating in the CD group. The IgG2 activity to gliadin varied much in CD and was 40-67% in 5 patients, while it was more uniform in the controls and never above 32%. Conversely, the main subclass activity to oat was found in IgG2 in both groups. Nearly all subclass activity to soya was IgG1 and IgG2 with the former dominating, except in two CD patients (70% and 95% IgG2). Treatment with a glutenfree diet usually reduced the IgG activity, but did not make great changes in the IgG-subclass proportions in 5 patients tested. The subclass pattern of individual patients may be of prognostic significance in CD. IgG1 and IgG3 antibodies activate complement, whereas IgG4 does not and shows minimal binding to Fc receptors on monocytes and lymphocytes. IgG4 may therefore block the phlogistic effect of IgG1 and IgG3. IgG4 may also block the binding of antigen to IgE on mast cells and basophils and thereby prevent release of amines. The high fraction of IgG2 antibodies to oat suggests that some CD patients may tolerate oat because this subclass does not activate complement. This possibility needs confirmation by controlled challenge of CD patients.

ISOLATION AND CHARACTERIZATION OF WHEAT PROTEINS WITH ANTIBODY REACTIVITY AGAINST SERUM OF A PATIENT WITH COELIAC DISEASE.

E. Molina, G. Gonzalez-Limas, J. Sequi, E.Mendez. Dep. of Endocrinology and Immunology. Hospital Ramon Y Cajal, Madrid, Spain.

An immunoblotting technique to identify gliadins reactive with antibodies of the serum from a coeliac child has been studied. Immunoblotting of a chloroform-methanol protein extract, (CM-extract), from wheat endosperm showed the presence of a considerable number of strong bands as well as a few weaker bands with relative molecular weight between 30 and 65 KD and between 10 and 25 KD respectively. The high molecular weight (HWM) components were well visualized using a wide range of the serum dilution, from 1/50 to 1/50000, while the fosfatase conjugated anti human Ig-A was kept at a dilution of 1/4000. Such bands were undetectable in a control immunoblotting using the serum of a healthy person when dilutions were higher than 1/1000. The CM-extract was separeted previously in two fractions by ammonium bicarbonate extraction. Analises by SDS-PAGE showed that most of the low molecular weight (LMW) components were found both in the soluble and insoluble bicarbonate fractions wheras the HMW-components were mainly localized in the latter. Both extracts were further fractionated by Reversed-Phase High Performance Liquid Chromatography, (rp-HPLC), using a semi-preparative Nucleosil C4 column. Immunoblotting analyses of the different fractions from the HPLC-chromatogram allowed the identification of about 6 to 10 HMW-components with elevated antigliadin antibody reactivities and 6 to 8 LMW-components with low reactivity. N-terminal sequences were determined by automatic sequencing of electroblotted proteins from the HPLC fractions into polyvinylidene-difluoride membranes. Since most of the LMW-components were N-terminal blocked, only three could be identified; the described as CM2 and CM3 and a new protein of about 23 KD which presents in the N-terminal region 37% homology with α-gliadin. Three different proteins of 35, 37 and 45 KD with the same N-terminal sequence than α-gliadin and another component of about 30 KD with nearly the same N-terminale sequence as δ-gliadin have been characterized from the HMW-components.

SPECIFIC IgA-GLIADIN ANTIBODY AS A MARKER OF RELAPSE IN COELIAC CHILDREN ON GLUTEN CHALLENGE.

C. Ribes-Koninckx, A. Ausina, C. Montero, M. Oltra, A. Pereda, J. Ferrer-Calvete.
Gastroenterological Unit. La Fe Children's Hospital - Valencia - Spain.

AIM: In order to assess the value of IgA Antigliadin antibody (IgA-AGA) measurement to predict mucosal relapse in coeliac children during a gluten challenge, a retrospective study on 65 children (Group I) and subsequently a prospective study on 25 children (Group II) was undertaken.

METHODS: Coeliac disease (CD) was confirmed according to ESPGAN criteria. Challenge consisted of 10 to 20 g gluten per day. Serum IgA-AGA were measured with an ELISA method already published. In group I, postchallenge biopsy was performed when clinical (even mild symptoms, such as failure to thrive or anorexia, were considered) or biochemical abnormality was detected with the following tests: d-xylose, low serum folate, Vit.B12 or iron levels, high serum IgA, or after 2 years on a gluten containing diet (GCD). In group II, biopsy was decided when high IgA-AGA were observed in two subsequent controls. IgA-AGA was measured after 1-3 months challenge and subsequently, controls were carried out every 3 months when normal IgA-AGA was found, or within one month when IgA-AGA was high.

RESULTS: Only 6 children (6/65=9.2%) in group I were biopsied within the first 6 months, and 35 (35/65=53.8%) at about 12 months. In 24 patients (24/65=36.9%) biopsy was performed after 2 years challenge, observing, in 2 of them, only minor changes in the mucosa; after one more year on a GCD, a severe villous atrophy was found in both. We found that these children had high IgA-AGA at the time of the first postchallenge biopsy; we also observed high IgA-AGA values in 72% children within the first year of the challenge period. Using IgA-AGA as an indication for biopsy, in group II, biopsy was indicated in 40% (10/25) of the children within the first 6 months and in 32% (8/25) between the 6th and the 12th month of the challenge period. In 4 cases with an early IgA-AGA control after 1 month on a GCD, biopsy was performed one month later. In 17 out of 18, a flat mucosa was found; one patient, with only minor changes in the mucosa, had a new biopsy performed 5 months later, confirming the diagnosis of CD. Only 1 patient had normal IgA-AGA after 2 years on a GCD; one year later a rise in IgA-AGA was detected, showing the mucosa a subtotal villous atrophy.

CONCLUSIONS: These results suggest that the period of gluten challenge can be considerably shortened when IgA-AGA mesurement is used in the follow up. Further studies are necessary at shorter intervals during gluten challenge to define the optimal period to perform the third confirmatory biopsy and avoid the deleterious effects of gluten in coeliac children.

GLUTEN AND DERMATITIS HERPETIFORMIS; CLINICAL OBSERVATIONS IN 5 ACTIVE DH PATIENTS ON AN ELEMENTAL DIET.

N. Zeedijk, J.B. van der Meer, H. Poen.
Depts of Dermatology Stadskanaal/ Emmen/Leeuwarden Depts of Gastroenterology Utrecht, The Netherlands.

Dermatitis Herpetiformis (DH) is a chronic and sometimes disabling itching vesiculobullous disease with a characteristic localization. Histological and immunopathological examination of skin biopsies showes highly specific pictures with sub epidermal microabcesses and granular IgA-deposition at the tips of the dermal papillae. Dapsone (diamino-diphenyl-sulfone) rapidly suppresses skin activity, however not without serious side-effects in higher doses. In some 80 to 90 % of DH patients histologically an enteropathy can be demonstrated identical with the villous atrophy in coeliac disease. The enteropathy is gluten-dependent as well. A gluten-free diet (GFD) improves the intestinal abnormalities concurrently with a decrease in skin activity, resulting in a lower minimal effective dose (MED) of Dapsone.
As to the pathogenesis of DH several authors propose an immunological mechanism by which circulating immune complexes, supposedly from intestinal origin, are deposited at the dermoepidermal junction, subsequently leading to micro-abcess formation.
As antigens evoking a humoral immuneresponse usually are proteins, it seems not unlogical to contribute an important role to dietary proteins in the formation of antigen-antibody complexes by the gut-associated lymfoid tissue. Gluten does not seem a likely candidate as a potential antigen, because it takes at least 5 months to more than a year before a GFD results in a gradual amelioration of skin condition.
To 5 active DH patients we administered an Elemental Diet (ED) (Variant 2000, Nutricia, Zoetermeer NL), thus eliminating dietary proteins totally.
In all patients a rapid improvement in skin condition occurred. This could not be attributed to gluten elimination, as some patients adhered to a strictly GFD more than a year preceding the study. Moreover in one patient simultaneous gluten challenge did not hamper the rapid beneficial effect of ED. In our opinion gluten only elevates the intestinal permeability which may facilitate the passage of antigens through the intestinal mucosa.

SERUM TRANSGLUTAMINASE IN THE FOLLOW-UP OF COELIAC DISEASE.

G. D'Argenio, R. Solazzo, I. Sorrentini, C. Ciacci, A. Gatto, P. Iovino, V. Cosenza, G. Mazzacca. Gastroenterology Unit, 2nd School of Medicine, University "Federico II", Napels - Italy.

Intestinal transglutaminase (TG) activity has been claimed to be involved in coeliac disease (CD) (1). A decreased serum TG activity in florid coeliac patients has recently been reported, while no significant differences were noted between treated coeliacs and controls (2). This presentation was a prospective study on serum TG changes in patients affected with CD. 10 Patients with CD diagnosed by routinary laboratory investigations and jejunal biopsy, were enrolledin this study. 5 Healthy volunteers, sex and age matched, made the control group. Serum TG was assaied by a radioenzymatic method (3) in untreated patients and after six months and 1 year of gluten free diet. The results are reported in the table. These results further support the finding of a decreased serum concentration of TG related to CD activity (2) and show the usefulness of serum TG assay either in the follow-up of CD and in monitoring gluten free diet responsiveness.

1 Bruce SE, Bjarnason I, Peters TJ, Clin.Sci. 1985, 68: 573-9
2 D'Argenio G et al. Gut 1989, 30: 950-954
3 Lorand L et al. Ann.Biochem. 1972, 50: 623-31

	Control subjects	Coeliac			
		Untreated	Treated (6 months)	Treated (1 year)	
Serum TG (mU/ml)		1.58±0.32 (p<0.001)	0.68±0.21 NS	1.24±0.33 NS	1.31±0.25

mU= 1 nmol of putrescine into acceptor protein at 37°C, pH=9.

METHODS FOR MEASUREMENT OF GLUTEN IN FOODSTUFFS

A.R. Freedman, H.J. Ellis, P.J. Ciclitira, Division of Pharmacology, UMDS, The Rayne Institute, St Thomas's Hospital, London, UK.

A gluten-free diet involves the avoidance of wheat, rye, barley and oats. Other cereals from the grass family graminae (eg maize and rice) are however, non-toxic to patients with coeliac disease. We wished to develop assays to measure coeliac toxic cereal proteins in foodstuffs. Whole gliadin was prepared from Kolibri strain wheat by the method of Patey & Evans (1973). The prolamin fractions from rye, barley, oats and maize were prepared by 70% ethanol extraction of their respective flours. Fifty mg/ml samples of test food stuffs were extracted with 70% ethanol. Unfractionated wheat gliadin was injected into New Zealand white rabbits to produce polyclonal antisera. The IgG fraction was purified by ammonium sulphate precipitation. Balb c mice were immunised with whole gliadin and their splenocytes fused with mouse myeloma cells, using standard techniques (Galfre & Milstein, 1981) ELISA asays were developed using polyclonal IgG as a capture antibody and mouse monoclonal antibody as the second antibody. Mouse monoclonal antibodies were used to develop immunodot binding assays.

The monoclonal ELISA showed low level cross-reactivity with rye, barley and oat prolamins, but none with non-toxic maize. Levels of 3.6 x 10-3, 3.3 x 10-3 and 2.0 x 10-2% by weight of gliadin were detected in nominally gluten-free products that are based on wheat starch. The immunodot binding assay gave qualitatively similar results with gliadin standards detectable at 10 μg/ml. Gliadin was detected in three nominally gluten-free flours. The prolamins from rye, barley and oats exhibited lower levels of cross-reactivitly, than gliadin. There was no cross-reaction with non-toxic maize. Monoclonal antibodies to wheat gliadin have been used to produce sensitive assays for the detection and quantitation of gliadin in foods for people with coeliac disease, particularly those that are nominally gluten-free but are based on wheat starch. The lower levels of cross-reaction of these assays with rye, barley and oat prolamins implies that it will not be possible to accurately screen all foodstuffs using a single assay until the coeliac toxic epitope has been indentified.

IDENTIFICATION OF COELIAC-ACTIVE PEPTIDES USING A NOVEL IN VITRO TEST FOR CELLULAR IMMUNITY

Jannine M. Devery and John H. Skerritt. CSIRO Wheat Research Unit, Division of Plant Industry, PO Box 7, North Ryde, NSW 2113, Australia.

The principal measurements of gluten hypersensitivity using coeliac blood samples have to date been the direct and indirect leucocyte migration inhibition factor assays (LMIF). The interaction of lymphokines with monocytes may also produce a membrane-bound procoagulant activity, which initiates coagulation to form a fibrin network around the cells, which restricts their movement. The production of macrophage procoagulant activity (MPCA) occurs with a concommitant decrease of the ability of cells to migrate from capillary tubes. As it is antigen-specific and has a direct correlation of delayed-type hypersensitivity skin test responses, MPCA has been proposed as an alternative measurement of cellular hypersensitivity in humans. We have thus used the test to identify coeliac-active peptides. In the MPCA peripheral blood mononuclear (PBM) cells are cultured with gluten anitgens, washed, and their ability to induce a procoagulant activity in normal platelet-poor plasma assessed either by measurement of prothrombin time or using a colorimetric assay. The basis of the assay is expression of thromboplastin receptors on macrophages which are induced by the antigen-specific lymphokine.

PBM from coeliac patients who had been on a gluten-free diet for less than two years responded strongly to gluten peptides, while coeliacs at diagnosis or who had maintained a strict gluten-free diet for longer than five years showed weaker responses. PBM from healthy volunteers did not respond to gluten or casein peptides, whereas those from patients with Crohn's disease displayed weak reactivity to both. Our study confirms previous findings that lymphoid cells from coeliacs exhibit a specific cellular immune response to gluten. This assay represents an alternative measure for cell-mediated immunity, is more sensitive and is technically much simpler than the LMIF assay. Macrophage procoagulant activity can either be measured using a simple plasma recalification time assay or spectrophotometrically using chromogenic substrates.

We have used both assays in detailed studies of the structural relationship between gliadin peptide sequence and coeliac activity. Firstly, we examined the role of the proline-serine-glutamine-glutamine (using the single letter amino acid code, PSQQ) motif on coeliac cellular immunity to gliadin derived-peptides, as this motif has been found in several large active peptides. Four peptides, corresponding to different regions of the alpha-gliadin molecule, were made by solid-phase derived synthesis. The sequence PSQQ (alone) was inactive because of its small size, while the peptide CPQPFPSQQPYLQ was very active. This peptide also contains the repeat-like motif QQPY, also found in gamma-gliadin and in rye and barley prolamins. Two other peptides, GSFRPSQQNPQAQG and CPQLQPNPSQQQPQEQ had zero and very slight activity respectively; they are surrounded by several charged amino acids and are thus distinct from much of the rest of the alpha-gliadin sequence. These sequences are also not found in gamma-gliadin. Secondly, several groups have developed algorithms which can predict likely T-cell epitopes. Certain of the key sequences present in the proline-poor gliadin region have been synthesised. However, none of these has shown activity in MPCA. It is likely therfore, that the coeliac active peptides are in the proline-rich N-terminal domain of gliadin sequences.

We wish to acknowledge the collaboration of Drs C Geczy and S Krilis.

UNRESPONSIVE SUBTOTAL VILLOUS ATROPHY, ULCERATIVE JEJUNITIS: TREATMENT WITH OMEPRAZOLE.

P.J. Kumar, M.L. Clark, A.M. Dawson. Dep. of Gastroenterology, St. Bartholomew's Hospital, UK.

A 45 year old man with subtotal villous atrophy unresponsive to a gluten-free diet and an elemental diet who developed ulcerative jejunitis. He was treated with omeprazole, prednisolone and azathioprine and is left with jejunal stricutures and small bowel dilatation. There is no evidence of lymphoma or any gene re-arrangement on antibody testing. A 45 year old man presented with a two year history of two stone weight loss and a a six week history of swollen legs and epigastric pain. There was a past history of recurrent iron deficiency anaemia. Investigation showed a haemoglobin of 15 g/dl, normal B12, low folates, an albumin of 17 g/l and raised faecal fats of 26 mmol in 24 hours. A jejunal biopsy showed subtotal villous atrophy and he was treated with a gluten-free diet (GFD). Over the next year he gained 15 kg in weight and his albumin rose to 44 g/l however, the barium follow trough remained unchanged with gross dilatation and coarse fold pattern and the jejunal biopsy showed some improvement. Subsequently, despite continuing a GFD his biopsy reverted to a subtotal villous atrophy pattern. He was therefore prescribed a diet omitting all bread and flour items including gluten-free following which he was given a six week course of elemental diet. As the biopsy remained unchanged after this the diagnosis of coeliac disease was questioned and he was therefore put on a normal diet. Within a week he presented with vomiting, epigastric pain, diarrhoea and feeling unwell. His temperature was 38.5°C, haemoglobulin 10.7 g/dl and the albumin had fallen to 22 g/l. He had lost 14 kg in weight. The barium follow through showed ulcerative jejunitis. He was therefore treated with total parenteral nutrition, omeprazole and hydrocortisone. In two weeks jejunoscopy showed that his ulceration had healed but the barium follow through now showed a stricture. A CT scan and ultrasound showed no abnormality and histology with monoclonal stains MTI, UCHI and Southern blots failed to show a lymphoma. In view of his vomiting he had a bypass operation but was left with a grossly dilated stomach and duodenal loop presumably due to further stricture formation. He is currently maintained on a GFD, omeprazole, steroids and azathioprine.

ACKNOWLEDGEMENTS

The organizers of the Dicke Symposium wish to thank the following institutions for their financial support:

. **Nutricia Nederland**
. Astra Pharmaceutical
. Byk Holland
. Dutch Foundation of Liver and Intestine
. Dutch Coeliac Society
. Dutch Ministry of Public Health and Culture
. E. Merck Holland
. Fisons Pharmaceutical
. FROSST/Merck, Sharp & Dohme
. Glaxo Production Group
. Gluten-free Products W. Sonneveld (Toseno)
. Gist Brocades Pharma Company PLC
. Juliana Children's Hospital
. M.S.D. Pharmaceutical
. Regionaal Ziekenfonds Twente
. Rorer Company PLC
. Smith Kline and Beecham
. Wilhelmina Children's Hospital
. Ziekenfonds Amersfoort en Omstreken
. Leiden University Hospital, Dept. of Paediatrics

All the editorial secretarial work was performed by:
Caroline de Vries-Kampschreur.
Dept. Hepatogastroenterology
Rijnstate Hospital
Arnhem - The Netherlands
Fax. 085 - 529275

Developments in Gastroenterology

1. A. S. Peña, I.T. Weterman, C.C. Booth and W. Strober (eds.): *Recent Advances in Crohn's Disease*. Proceedings of the 2nd International Workshop on Crohn's Disease, held in Noordwijk/Leiden, The Netherlands (1980). 1981 ISBN 90–247–2475–9
2. P.M. Motta and L.J.A. Didio (eds.): *Basic and Clinical Hepatology*. 1982 ISBN 90–247–2404–X
3. D. Rachmilewitz (ed.): *Inflammatory Bowel Diseases*. Proceedings of the 1st International Symposium, held in Jerusalem, Israel (1981). 1982 ISBN 90–247–2612–3
4. D. Fleischer, D. Jensen and P. Bright-Asare (eds.): *Therapeutic Laser Endoscopy in Gastrointestinal Disease*. 1983 ISBN 0–89838–577–6
5. S.P. Borriello (ed.): *Antibiotic Associated Diarrhoea and Colitis*. The Role of *Clostridium difficile* in Gastrointestinal Disorders. 1984 ISBN 0–89838–623–3
6. Ch.H. Gips and R.A.F. Krom (eds.): *Progress in Liver Transplantation*. 1985 ISBN 0–89838–726–4
7. G.F. Nelis, J. Boevé and J.J. Misiewicz (eds.): *Peptic Ulcer Disease: Basic and Clinical Aspects*. Proceedings of a Symposium on Peptic Ulcer Today, held at the Sophia Ziekenhuis, Zwolle, The Netherlands (1984). 1985 ISBN 0–89838–759–0
8. D. Rachmilewitz (ed.): *Inflammatory Bowel Diseases 1986*. Proceedings of the 2nd International Symposium, held in Jerusalem, Israel (1985). 1986 ISBN 0–89838–796–5
9. E.M.H. Mathus-Vliegen: *The Role of Laser in Gastroenterology*. Analysis of Eight Years' Experience. 1989 ISBN 0–7923–0425–X
10. D.M. Jensen and J.-M. Brunetaud (eds.): *Medical Laser Endoscopy*. 1990 ISBN 0–7923–0579–5
11. D. Rachmilewitz and J. Zimmerman (eds.): *Inflammatory Bowel Diseases 1990*. Proceedings of the 3rd International Symposium, held in Jerusalem, Israel (1989). 1990 ISBN 0–7923–0657–0
12. L. Capocaccia, G. Ricci, F. Angelico, M. Angelico, A.F. Attili and L. Lalloni (eds.): *Recent Advances in the Epidemiology and Prevention of Gallstone Disease*. Proceedings of the 2nd International Workshop, held in Rome, Italy (1989). 1991 ISBN 0-7923-0994-4
13. M.L. Mearin and C.J.J. Mulder (eds.): *Coeliac Disease*. 40 years gluten free. 1991 ISBN 0-7923-1160-4

Kluwer Academic Publishers – Dordrecht / Boston / London